"Wow—what a perfect combination: Eric and Max! A book on general fitness by this incredible team could change a person's life. It's fascinating to just hear them talk about how the body responds to training. It is very motivating to work with people who genuinely care about what they are doing."

—Jim Ochowicz
founder, general manager, and coach of 7-Eleven cycling team from 1981 through 1990

"I was a guy who could compete at the state level—until I started working with Max. In a little more than a year, I was national champion, and placed in the top ten in the world two years in a row."

—Warren Geissart, 49
weekend cycling racer
national sprint champion

"Max and Eric are both remarkable resources for the sports, science, and medical communities and two of the most down-to-earth people I have ever met. When it comes to actually practicing the art of applying science and medicine to human activity, they are an unbeatable combination."

—Steve Johnson
president, USA Cycling

"When I have a training question, Eric is the first person I go to after my coach. I always know Eric is going to give a different perspective to me. What Eric accomplished is probably the most amazing feat in Olympic history. We look up to him like he's a god."

—Chad Hedrick
Olympic speed skater

"The abilities of Eric Heiden and Max Testa combine to create a synergy of world-class forces. Dr. Testa is a walking encyclopedia on physiological theory and Dr. Heiden is a living inspiration on effectively applying those theories. They have helped my athletes to achieve Olympic medals and world records, but even more than that, they have helped my athletes to go beyond what we thought possible."

—Tom Cushman
U.S. speed-skating coach

"I thought I was at the top of my abilities. I was eighth and ninth in the Tour de France, and I was wondering if that was as good as I could get. I started working with Max, and I've improved like I never thought I would. I'm at a different level now."

—Levi Leipheimer
3rd place, 2007 Tour de France
Deseret Morning News, Oct. 4, 2007

"In the fall of 1990, the six-foot-two-inch Spanish rider [Miguel Indurain] weighed a muscular 184 pounds—too heavy to stay competitive in the mountain stages of the Tour de France. But that winter, a consultant to Indurain's team, Max Testa, figured out the optimal ratio of power to body weight for cyclists, based on his studies of past Tour winners. To reach it, Indurain had to shed only 12 pounds. Which he did. The next year he won his first of five consecutive Tours [de France]."

Outside Magazine, Feb. 2005

"Max Testa is phenomenal—I've never known anyone who is as good at taking text-book theory and breaking it down into usable pieces which you can easily and effectively fit into a real training program."

—Tom Cushman
U.S. speed-skating coach

"Massimo Testa was the key to all of my successes for my entire 12-year career as a pro racer. He and I happened to have turned to professional cycling the same day, at the '85 Giro d'Italia. He was fresh out of medical training, I was scraping the North Dakota dirt off my shoes determined to make it as a pro in Europe. As naive as I was fresh to pro racing I had strong suspicions about doping in pro racing and was determined to avoid it at all costs. I have to admit I had no use for a "Team Doctor" due to my prejudices. Max impressed me first as an honest man of impeccable morals worthy of the title doctor, and then as the best ally I could ever hope for to keep me healthy, strong, superbly trained, and in a state of relaxed hunger for victories. None of my wins would have happened without Max's guidance."

—Andy Hampsten
winner of the '88 Giro d'Italia, '86 and '87 Tours of Switzerland,
4th at the Tour de France in '86 and '92

"Max came to our team with humor and a straightforward approach to cycling sports medicine. He calmed the nerves and fears of the team riders as we had just entered the ranks of professional cycling. Max understood rider psychology and knew how to get the best out of each of us. It was always great to have Max around the team because he knew how to keep things in perspective. He was the reason I lived in Como during my pro career in Europe."

—Ron Kiefel
seven-time Tour de France competitor, 1984 Olympic bronze medalist, the first
American to win a stage in the Giro d'Italia, and owner of the legendary
Wheat Ridge Cyclery in Wheat Ridge, Colorado

"Max and Eric are experts in their field, but they are also two of the nicest, most down-to-earth people I have ever met. Together it seems they are capable of solving almost any problem an athlete might have, whether it's a training problem or a medical problem. It's rare to find people like Max and Eric, and when you do, I think it's very beneficial to listen to what they have to say."

—Dave Zabriskie
elite U.S. national time trial champion

"Twenty-five years later, Eric Heiden is still a legend within long-track speed skating. He trained at a different level, had a different mind-set, and did something in the sport that probably will never be done again. What he did was simply amazing. He achieved the impossible. Fifty years from now his dominance in the sport will still be remembered."

—Apolo Anton Ohno
speed-skating gold medalist

"With Team 7-Eleven, Max and Eric started having them do intervals while everyone else was riding 5 hours a day. Other coaches laughed at them—until they won a stage in the Giro, and then the Tour de France. It still happens today. They've developed unconventional techniques, based on their knowledge of medicine, while other coaches persist in staying with what is traditional."

—Warren Geissart
weekend cycling racer

"I have always been amazed by Eric's intensity, fitness, and drive and now he has got it all in a book so that everyone can reach their fitness goals. Well done!"

—John McEnroe

"Any physician who works with people looking to regain the health and energy of their younger days knows exercise is the answer, and this book is the prescription for it. It's as if they read the minds of every doctor who has wondered how to get people moving the *right* way and wrote this book to make fitness a real possibility for everyone."

—Sean Degnan, M.D.

"For those of us with day jobs, this program shows how much more efficient you can be with your training time. Every minute has a purpose; within a month or two I could feel the effects. I felt enormous improvement—and it all came after many years of training. I just wish I'd done the program when I was 23! But I can't complain, at 40 I feel as fast as I've ever been."

—Tad Borek
investment adviser, amateur athlete

"As a women's health physician, and running coach to hundreds of beginner runners, it is refreshing to see a book that addressed not just elite athletes but those who are just beginning. By allowing a layperson a bird's-eye view into the science behind exercise, the health benefits of physical activity are now within everyone's reach!"

Karen H. Zufelt, MD
founder of RunningForWomen.com

"Drawing on their decades of experience, two of the most-respected and best-liked people in bicycle racing have collaborated on this easy-to-follow, sensible guide to a healthier life. Max Testa and Eric Heiden say all it will take is 12 weeks. What are you waiting for?"

—Samuel Abt, author of *Breakaway* and
LeMond, former associate editor of the
International Herald and contributor to the
New York Times

faster, better, stronger

faster, better, stronger

Your Exercise Bible, for a Leaner, Healthier Body in Just 12 Weeks

ERIC HEIDEN, M.D.,

MASSIMO TESTA, M.D.,
and DeAnne Musolf

HARPER

NEW YORK • LONDON • TORONTO • SYDNEY

HARPER

Photographs used in conjunction with stretching exercises featured in Part Two used with permission by Brooks Stevenson, Intermountain Healthcare.

FIRST HARPER PAPERBACK PUBLISHED 2009.

Designed by Meryl Sussman Levavi

The Library of Congress has catalogued the hardcover edition as follows:

Heiden, Eric.
    Faster, better, stronger : 10 proven secrets to a healthier body in 12 weeks / By Eric Heiden and Massimo Testa; and DeAnne Musolf.—1st ed.
        p. cm.
    Includes bibliographical references.
    ISBN 978-0-06-121523-0
1. Physical fitness. I. Testa, Massimo. II. Musolf, DeAnne. III. Title.

RA781.H378 2008
613.7—dc22

2008002582

ISBN 978-0-06-121529-2 (pbk.)

09 10 11 12 13 WBC/RRD 10 9 8 7 6 5 4 3 2 1

To Connor, Zoe, and Karen. You are the best.
—E.H.

To Julie, Sara, and Marco
—M.T.

To Ryan, and to Tony
—D.M.

contents

acknowledgments

There are many people whom I would like to thank. I feel that I should start with my parents, Tina and Matteo Testa, for teaching me the value of a good education. A very special thank you goes to my wife, Julie, and our children, Sara and Marco, for their love and understanding during my years of traveling around the world for yet another big bike tour.

During my career working with athletes, a few people made a difference in determining my focus on exercise and health. One of these was my mentor, Professor Renzo Minelli, M.D., who taught me the interesting field of exercise physiology, and the superior value of preventing rather than curing disease. Another special person is Jim Ochowicz, who in 1985 gave me support and my first opportunity to apply training science to his professional cycling team. I am also really grateful to Eric Heiden for his friendship of over twenty years. Because of his vision of a comprehensive sports medicine program, I was able to start a new chapter of life in the United States. This book comes as a result of our collaboration and a common vision of considering every athlete a special one. However, this book would never have happened without the contribution of DeAnne Musolf, who gave words in an organized sequence to our working experiences. Thank you, DeAnne, for your hard work.

I also would like to thank my working partners at TOSH, within the Department of Sport Science and Medicine, and the Department of Physical Therapy and Rehabilitation. Every day I learn something from them.

To conclude, I would like to thank all my patients and athletes who trusted me with their varied challenges. I always felt that what I learned from them was more valuable than what I was able to give.

—MASSIMO TESTA, M.D.

I would like to acknowledge those who came before us and discovered the foundation of knowledge we use every day to help our patients and clients, those who allowed us to contribute and participate in their athletic success, and Max for being a good friend and professional colleague.

—Eric Heiden, M.D.

I am grateful to Max and Eric for allowing me the privilege of working with them to bring this valuable information to light. You are truly great human beings, not to mention kind, funny, very talented, and wise. Your genius in this field is only outsized by your tremendous care for other people.

Kathy Huck, thank you for your expert guidance. You really knew how to get to the heart of the matter and this book is so much the better for it. Thank you, Helen Song, for your stellar attitude and your great work. We also extend our appreciation to the other members of our team at Harper-Collins: Matthew Benjamin, Teresa Brady, Angie Lee, Cassandra Gonzalez, and Meryl Sussman Levari. Thanks to each of you for your superb efforts on this book. Farley Chase, thanks for believing in this.

To the extraordinarily insightful Anthony Guffanti, without whom I might still be looking for a worthwhile book project and Eric and Max might still be dreaming of doing a book someday.

I am on my knees with gratitude to the brilliant and insightful reader, writer, and dear friend Em Yates, who likened my writing this book (while doing two other jobs and single parenthood) to Ginger Rogers, who danced as well as Fred Astaire, "but backward and wearing high heels." Thank you, Em, for your generous spirit. And to Gina Simmerling for her heroic efforts to bring fitness to the world through *Active Cities* magazine, and to Ashley Simpson and Elise Marton for their fabulous editing and support while also dancing backward in high heels, to Sara Hare for her sage advice, and to Julie Dow and Amy Raymond for their tireless assistance when I needed it. To my mother, Janice Nephew, for her fantastic faith, good spirits, and love; to Tammi Musolf for her expert insight into health matters and her never-ending energy and enthusiasm for my ideas; and to Jamee Klosters and Beth Yates for their lifelong friendship. All of you have shown me all that women can do.

We are also indebted to experts Mike Lardon, M.D., Marlia Braun, Ph.D., and Fran Mason, M.D., for their amazing work and invaluable contributions to our motivation, nutrition, and sleep content respectively, and to artist Kat Weiss, for bringing a bit of beauty to our otherwise plain pages. All kind and smart people.

Julie Testa, thanks to you, too. Every time I see you I am in awe; I want to shake your hands—all eight of them. To Sara and Marco Testa, thanks for the Ping-Pong, biking, and bubble blowing between work sessions, and the enchanting Connor, Zoe, and Karen Heiden for letting me come and stay in your wonderful, warm home.

I also want to acknowledge the substantial influence of my father, Bertram Musolf, who with my mother's help was committed to daily exercise and a low-fat diet long before it was fashionable. In northern Minnesota, if you were out for a run in those days, people pulled over and offered you a ride. Though he died when I was only eight years old, Dad's love of exercise and the outdoors unhindered by rain, blizzards, darkness, cold, a 9–5 job, and myriad logistics shaped my life.

Last, I want to acknowledge the person who makes my life a joyful adventure today: Ryan, my six-year-old son, who also constantly works my flexibility, strength, and cardiovascular system.

Ryan said to me the other day, "I love you, Mom, all the way to Neptune and back a million times," which astonished me, because this is exactly how much I love him.

—DeAnne Musolf

introduction

THE TALE OF TWO DOCTORS

In the last few decades, there has been explosive growth in exercise science. We have witnessed it as doctors and in our own athletic endeavors, huffing around speed-skating rinks and bounding up Alpe d'Huez and—more important—helping others do it. We offer this book as a means of spreading those discoveries.

People continually come to us with the same questions about exercise, repeated tales of wasted months and years without the fitness or the health they sincerely seek. It's not for lack of trying. Millions slave away at one-size-fits-all fitness programs, not even tailoring them to their individual exercise needs. Many don't even know they *have* individual needs. And people in general, no matter their starting level, are overwhelmed by misconceptions about exercise heaped upon them, few of which are based on medical reality. Sadly, we see people spend time, energy, and money committing the same training errors.

Before coming to us, that is.

Our experience is that people are genuinely eager to exercise, and that they can be disciplined and effective—if they know where to start and exactly what to do; they need a fitness philosophy that works, that they can embrace for life. So what works? Herein lies the problem. People who know exercise science and people who exercise never talk to one another. Most doctors read only medical journals, and not much about training science, while sports scientists who develop and analyze training research often don't work with individual athletes. And if people see a sports doctor at all, it's for an injury, not for training advice. So relatively little of the great techniques developed by exercise scientists ever reaches people who exercise. Instead, fitness-seekers get training advice from a nurse they know from the gym, from a trainer certified online (which we would caution against—many athletic training certification sites require only a fee, no course work or testing), or from a brief list of tips, and none with respect to their current condition. Or people exercise the way they always did, based on what their coach told them to do in high school.

It became clear to us that some of the training programs currently available, though wildly popular, are wanting in terms of very basic facts. We know that everyone who wants fitness deserves a lot better, and they get a lot better when they have good information.

We study exercise science *and* we work with people who exercise. We have coaxed many athletes into the new, science-based era of fitness. Medically, we know how training works, and we know what information fitness-seekers need to make it work in the real world. We keep up on continuing research—there remains much to be learned, but we also know far more than we did ten, even five years ago. In our athletes and in our patients, we've seen the metamorphosis that occurs when the lightbulb goes on regarding how exercise actually works.

First, research shows us that an effective exercise program needs to pinpoint each individual's starting point. Ours does. In addition, studies show that the best programs also need to be tailored to a broad range of starting abilities. Ours also does that. We are veterans of the fitness battlefield; we know the best strategies for victory with new recruits as well as the celebrated and the battle weary. We know the training needs and goals of beginners as intimately as those of elite athletes, and we respectfully address the entire spectrum and acknowledge individual differences.

Second, the right information needs to be geared for the general public. Our program is unique in that it is designed for everyday people. Unlike many fitness programs, it doesn't rely on knowledge gleaned from helping beautiful people stay beautiful; it's not based on what worked for people who are already in good shape, who are well disposed to stay in good shape, and who have ready access to swimming pools and gyms and are not stuck in an office all day. Too often, everyday people "mysteriously" fail when they try those programs. We know that the luxuries of time and access are significant factors in getting fit. Just about everyone could easily be fit if they had a staff, were paid to be fit, and didn't have a job and a family. *Faster, Better, Stronger* is, instead, based on what we have seen works for *every*one who wants to get in shape, people who work and have a family or other obligations, who don't necessarily have a gym membership or four hours a day to work out or plan meals.

We understand, because we too have day jobs. We work as physicians, with Olympians and everyday athletes, with people you see at the grocery store, and with people you see on professional teams. In fact, we developed the UC Davis Sports Performance Program because we wanted to give every fitness-seeker a place to go for sports orthopedic, nutrition, physiological, biomechanical, and psychological guidance under one roof, to establish a place where sports medicine could be tendered in a more comprehensive, holistic way. Our facility has blossomed into one of the premier training centers in the United States. Since then, we have expanded our vision to Utah's The Orthopedic Specialty Surgery Hospital (TOSH), whose goals reflect ours: to be the best sports medicine and injury prevention facility in the world, and one of the few in the country to open its doors to athletes from seasoned pro to newcomer. This hospital and sports research center, where Eric works as both a surgeon and the medical director, offers surgery, rehab, human performance testing and coaching programs, nutrition consultation, bone density testing, motion analysis, pool therapy, and more—a veritable candy store for anyone who's ever wondered about exercise and his or her body. Much of what we supply in this book mirrors advice we prescribe to clients at TOSH, based on the training philosophy we have developed over decades.

We have helped people of all athletic abilities achieve their best, based on their goals. Some of them ended up winning national and international titles. Others happily finished their first century bike ride or 5k walk.

It all started in 1985 when Massimo Testa, M.D. (or Max as friends call him), became team physician for the 7-Eleven professional cycling team. We didn't know it then, but this American team would usher U.S. cyclists into the international spotlight for the first time. Team 7-Eleven with team manager Jim Ochowicz (now USA Cycling president) and team director Mike Neel (the first American to ride for a Europe-based team) was also a "Who's Who" of people who would go on to become cycling legends: Andy Hampsten (the first and only American to win the Giro d' Italia—the Italian version of the Tour de France), Bob Roll (currently a Tour de France commentator), Davis Phinney (a Tour de France stage winner and author of one of the classic books on cycling), Chris Carmichael (who went on to train Lance Armstrong), Ron Kiefel (the first American to win a stage in the Giro), Tom Schuler (one of the most successful cycling and sports managers of all time), Jonathan Boyer (the first American to race in the Tour de France, and a two-time winner of the Race Across America), Jeff Bradley (a national champion multiple times and currently a successful bike shop owner in Iowa), and Jeff "Peppy"

Pierce (the first American to win the final stage of the Tour de France in Paris). And then there was Eric Heiden.

Eric was twenty-five years old. Five years earlier, at the Winter Olympic Games in Lake Placid, New York, he had won all five men's speed-skating races. After he had retired from speed skating and started medical school, he turned to another passion of his—cycling—and joined Team 7-Eleven.

Together, we observed that the team's cyclists did not enjoy the benefits of scientific exercise training. (Even today, in the United States, sports medicine is not a preventative medical specialty focused on exercise science and performance as it is in Europe.) Eric had been exposed to a scientific approach to exercise training as a skater. Max had studied training science as part of his specialty as a medical student in Italy, applying structured, individualized training to all kinds of athletes from amateurs to professionals. In contrast, 7-Eleven cyclists' daily program focused mainly on volume, without the full benefit of the structure or organization we knew advanced performance. Their approach was to simply ride, and ride hard, but without a plan, a target, or a goal, and without distinguishing between the various types of fatigue. The team's cyclists displayed great enthusiasm and discipline, but to us they seemed miles from reaching their potential, and many were essentially pedaling up the wrong road.

We convinced some of our teammates to try a more structured training approach. With that, this program was born.

For American pro cycling, it was a pivotal moment. Ours was a unique combination of athletic experience and cutting-edge sports medicine knowledge. With it, Team 7-Eleven went on to astonish the European cycling world with stage wins in the Giro d'Italia and Tour de France. It gradually shifted the axis of American professional cycling, and this is reflected in America's showings in the international arena today. A young and talented Lance Armstrong joined the team and won the world championship in 1993, and the rest is history.

This information is simple, but may represent a turning point for you as well. Even if you feel you have read everything on fitness that has come down the track, *Faster, Better, Stronger* will help you look at your training in a different way. This program does not make for quick sound bites, however; it can't be summed up in an advertising blurb, and it's not based on what worked for one supermodel or high-profile athlete. We don't simplify proven training techniques to make you feel like you have really "gotten something," only to frustrate you when you try to actually use it.

Nor does our information require a calculator and a degree in exercise physiology to understand. Instead, it's plain-speak on what people need to know to get fit, based on what has worked scientifically, in hundreds of cases. And we present it in a way that's easy to understand and simple to do—we're good at that. We explain things to people who seek better fitness every day. We believe that taking the time to do so makes a positive difference in the outcome. We also think we have quite a bit of experience at making real exercise science doable for everyone.

We have one confession to make: The information in this book is really no secret. Olympians and elite athletes in Europe practice these methods; the coaches who train them know about these techniques and so do the scientists who have proven what works. Every one of them knows one piece of the puzzle or another. Almost all of the components of our approach have already been written up in medical journals squirreled away in the recesses of your public library. We did not create these techniques. The problem is that those elite athletes and their trainers are reluctant to reveal what they know, owing to the fact that their livelihood depends upon maintaining an edge over the competition. The scientists who publish in the medical journals don't directly train real people. And real people rarely want to spend their time at the library poring over stuffy medical journals. We are not bound by any of these constraints. We follow training science and have applied it. We, in essence, close the loop.

The knowledge in this book encapsulates forty years of our accumulated reading of scientific and medical journals combined with as many years of our practical experience at world championships, the grand European bike tours, and the Olympic Games, center stage and behind the scenes. We have assembled all of the pieces of the training puzzle, fitted them together to form the big picture, and then tested it in the real world. Now we want you to benefit, to use it to enrich your health with every stride, dance step, or pedal stroke.

With this information, there is no reason for you to spend another breath or another dime on outmoded training techniques. The time has come to bring your exercise methods into the new millennium. For us, the true measure of our success is how many people we reach with this information.

In Part One of this book, we detail the solid science behind your body's responses to exercise. Humans are thinking animals; we do better at *anything* when we understand how and why it works. So we give you scientific "secrets" in several areas of fitness: the prescriptive aspects of exercise; the kinds of movement your body needs; how to get started; how you improve as you move; fueling your body with the right food and water; what rest really accomplishes; how to buy and use gear properly and avoid injuries; and motivation. These "secrets" can help you throughout your life and can be applied to any exercise program, be it ours or another you try. We shepherd you around medically known fitness pitfalls; we also debug and clarify some all-too-often-misunderstood medical and biological truths about exercise. We offer you ways to find your hidden talents and strengths (yes, we all have them) and to compensate with intelligence and mental focus for the gaps in natural ability (which we also all have).

In Part Two of this book, we help you design your own unique, individualized exercise program based on the marriage of scientific outcomes and what we've seen works on the street and in the gym. We know that everyone's biology is a little different, and each person has a unique constellation of strengths and weaknesses. For this reason, Part Two begins with several easy self-assessments (or optional lab tests) in four areas: cardiovascular endurance, strength, flexibility, and coordination. Once you have assessed your current fitness level, we guide you through assembling blocks of activities into a twelve-week program. Beginners and those at risk start with sessions of very light exercise, fitter readers with more rigorous exercise. No matter your condition now, you will precisely customize the intensity of your exercise sessions and their duration to increase your level of fitness as you progress through the twelve weeks. Each week of exercise is broken into very doable daily blocks of twenty to sixty minutes each. Each block concentrates on one or more of the basic components of fitness. We also give you the means to adjust the program to fit you exactly, based not on intuition, the hottest new training technique, or what your best friend does, but on exercise science. We then give you instructions on how to recalibrate your exercise for another twelve weeks, and onward in your new life of fitness. We also offer activities, exercises, and workout routines for you to use to accelerate your progress. These concepts are similar to those we originally designed for our clients, many of whom are professional athletes.

In this manner, *Faster, Better, Stronger* focuses your time and attention on precisely what works and what's necessary *for you*. This program isn't designed just for jocks, and it doesn't take much time. An investment of four to eight hours per week (for most people) could add immeasurable quality to your life; with it you could become more active, vital, and energetic, and more likely to live free from disease, pain, and medication. This is a customized, science-based program designed to guide you into a life-long fitness habit, a life during which you can feel more alive, eat better, sleep more soundly, age more gracefully, work more efficiently, be mentally sharper, play harder, and feel happier.

So you want to get more fit? Feel healthier, be stronger, look younger, live longer? You can. We will show you how. We will give you step-by-step instructions on how to make the most of your body through exercise—physically, mentally, biomechanically, and nutritionally. We have seen good, substantial outcomes—harder abs, lower cholesterol, and leaner bodies—and you will, too.

Your success will depend in part upon teaming up with a physician. You wouldn't take your car on a cross-country journey without having it first given a thumbs-up by a mechanic. In our experience, many of us have our cars checked more often than we do our own bodies. So talk to your doctor. Take your body in for a checkup and have your major systems tested before you begin this journey. Even a small change in activity can have broad and highly individual consequences. Doctors are not Merlin, and modern diagnostic equipment is not a crystal ball, but physicians do have special expertise and technology that enable them to detect problems that are silent or invisible to the naked eye. And they can often help you fix them or avoid breakdowns with simple adjustments to your exercise plan. Call your doctor and explore with her how a fitness plan might affect you.

Sharing how exercise affects people, in fact, inspired us to write this book. By doing that we hope to benefit what is perhaps the organ most important to your overall fitness: your brain.

—Eric Heiden, M.D.
—Max Testa, M.D.

how
and why

"Our bodies are our gardens, our wills our gardeners."
—William Shakespeare

1

better shape

When you buy a car, you know that it will slowly deteriorate the more you use it. Park it in a garage and it will remain pristine, but drive it and the tires will wear out, its oil will need changing, its paint will grow dull, and its working parts will break down. Put more miles on a compact and it does not become a Mercedes or a Ferrari.

Your body, however, is different. It *does* become a Ferrari the more you use it. How? We have arrived at ten requirements, or secrets, to making that happen. These basic tenets, listed here and explained in the coming chapters, are guaranteed to usher you to greater fitness. If you follow these general rules, *you will get better.*

1. **Follow the right program.** Choose a program that is scientifically based and can be tailored to your needs. Then stick with that program for at least twelve weeks.
2. **Set a goal**. The right main objective along with certain incremental goals provides the perfect mix of mile markers and motivation.
3. **No patience, no gain.** Gauge your expectations for achieving your goals not by the clock, as you would a salon treatment, but by the calendar, as you would a vegetable garden.
4. **Assess your starting point.** To get from Point A to Point B, you have to find out your current condition—your Point A.
5. **Alternate hard and easy days, working on not just one but all four**

components of fitness: aerobic conditioning, strength training, flexibility, and balance and coordination.

6. **Treat exercise like the powerful drug that it is.** "Take" your exercise at the right time, in the right amount and intensity, for the right duration.

7. **Fuel your body with the right food and fluids.** Eat from all of the food groups, and at the right times (especially before, during, and after exercise), to provide the ideal building blocks your body requires for fitness.

8. **Equip yourself with the right basic gear and troubleshoot aches and pains early.** Doing this can go a long way in helping you go a long way.

9. **Train your brain.** Know the vast physiological metamorphosis exercise sets in motion in your body. Your positive (or negative) thoughts and your understanding of what's happening with your body have a motivational *and* a biological impact.

10. **Everyone can get better.** *Everyone.*

These ten concepts encapsulate what we have witnessed working when it comes to the discipline of fitness. If you read no further but apply these rules to any program you use from now on, you will have already notched up your ability to hone your body through exercise. We'll show you how to apply these rules in the rest of this chapter and throughout the book.

Follow the Right Program

We live in the most fitness-conscious civilization ever known. The proliferation of gyms, popular exercise regimens, videos, and yoga studios has made fitness a multimillion-dollar business and has sustained a variety of fitness philosophies, many in conflict with one another. Millions of people spend too much time, money, and sweat to get fit, and often they fail. Why? They suffer from the same debilitating fitness problem: oversimplified approaches and techniques, often explained by people with limited medical or scientific background.

Too many of these fitness ideas are based on one piece of scientific understanding and not the whole picture. They address only one facet of fitness, or they address all of us as if we were so many identical widgets marching out of a factory with the same strengths and weaknesses, the same starting point, and the same schedule. "Experts" of the moment oblige everyone's desire for fitness information. They dish out advice that is loosely based on a technique that worked for a few celebrities or one high-profile athlete; thus a "hot new training tip" starts circulating. Would-be athletes instantly feel that they have been given some secret to achieving higher performance . . . until they start applying it. Then they realize they have nothing. And they fail again.

The sheer number of magic fitness tricks out there tells you there's no magic trick. Magic? No. But there is an entire field of training science and medicine relatively unknown to the average fitness-seeker. So we will give you an exercise plan, yes, but also the proven science that is the basis of the plan. We will give you "what to do" but also "why to do it," backed by a huge body of evidence, which is the root of our guarantee: You can definitely get more fit. Once you understand the how and why, you will be armed for fitness for the rest of your life.

Why a Program?

So why do you need a program? Why not just do a lot of everything?

If you moved to a part of the world where there were no cars, no escalators, no UPS—say, to the steppes of Mongolia—maybe you wouldn't need an exercise program. Or if you lived in a society where your lifestyle required a great range of daily physical activity, again, maybe you wouldn't need a program. Certainly preceding generations did not. But because the amount of activity required of most people today is so minimal, and the time available to exercise is so tightly circumscribed by work, family, civic, and other obligations, most people need to be precise with the precious time they do commit to fitness.

Fitness is a term that encompasses a fistful of physical qualities: cardiovascular health, muscular strength, flexibility, balance and coordination, and ideal weight. A person who is fit, in our mind, embodies all of these qualities. To help you get there while making the best use of your exercise time, money, and energy, our fitness program proposes the best activities at the correct duration and intensity, a week at a time.

Each week of this program is a cocktail of varying activities, thirty to sixty minutes in length. A typical week looks something like this:

Tuesday	Wednesday	Thursday	Friday	Saturday	Sunday	Monday
Aerobic	Flexibility + Strength	Aerobic	Flexibility + Aerobic	Aerobic + Strength	Aerobic	Rest

We prescribe to patients the exact duration and intensity of activity they need each day, but those specifications would be hieroglyphics to you now if we listed them here. By the time you reach Part Two, however, it will be a piece of cake. There we will shepherd you through assembling the ideal twelve-week program for *you*, based on your current level of fitness.

SET A GOAL

Reasonable long-term and incremental goals, we have found, aren't necessarily for the good days, but for the bad days. Any one of a number of goals may be the trigger that gets you out the door. But a goal is only effective if it's the right goal—not too easily attainable and not too lofty. People come into our clinic who have never exercised but want to buy a bike. This is good. Then they will say, "My goal is to do the Death Ride," a popular California event that includes 16,000 feet of climbing over 130 miles. And they want to do it in, say, three months. We give our athletes every tool we've got to help them achieve their goals, but such relatively high aspirations require that the body be given time to build the systems necessary to do it. This type of short-term goal is a setup for failure, though it might be appropriate as a long-term goal.

NO PATIENCE, NO GAIN

Many people we see also have weight loss as a goal. The dual ambitions of losing weight *and* gaining fitness require more careful attention to the plan, because you need to consume enough calories to fuel vigorous exercise and healthy recovery while simultaneously keeping a precise negative caloric balance in order to lose weight. The good news is that you can lose weight while getting fit, but these two things don't happen in three months, or in six months. They require precise steps along a carefully laid path.

We advocate the minimum number of hours at the lowest (easiest) intensity possible to see gain, yes, but the considerable physical metamorphosis caused by exercise takes time. People want to lose ten pounds in ten minutes; they think of a workout at the gym like a visit to a hair salon: They walk in, do their time, and expect to walk out transformed. They go for a bike ride and weigh themselves when they get home to see if they've lost weight. People think fitness should be satisfying in the same manner as buying new clothes or a new gadget; they anticipate instant gratification. There are gratifying facets of fitness that do come quickly—some, such as the pure pleasure you feel for the rest of the day, are immediate—but the seeds of immense long-term change must first be sown, then grown. Fitness is cultivated on the same scale as a garden—over a season, not overnight.

ASSESS YOUR STARTING POINT

What has put this exercise program in the winner's circle time and again is that it provides each individual athlete with the tools to focus his time and energy precisely where *he* needs it, for as long as *he* needs it. It's a tailored program of maximum benefit for minimum output, requiring as little as four hours a week for twelve weeks.

Everyone in the human race has different strengths biologically. Think of all the people you know as if they represent the various specialties of track and field: Some folks are light but can't go fast; some are ideal for shot put, others for the high jump or the javelin; some for sprints and others for distance. You have your own strengths, and you need to pinpoint them and leverage them to get fit. Fitness is not all or nothing, on or off. It's a spectrum—at one extreme are the athletes who are very good at one thing, in the middle are people who are average in all the components, and at the other extreme are people with the most to gain.

In Part Two you will test yourself in each area, starting with your cardiovascular health. Based on your starting point in aerobic fitness combined with your risk factors, you will be "prescribed" an aerobic exercise intensity that will make the best use of your time as you begin your program. We will also give you a way to gauge the heat—or intensity—of your exercise. This assessment will allow you to take advantage of your strengths and rev up your weaknesses. The amount of aerobic, flexibility, and muscular strength training you will do each week depends upon your score in each of those areas. You will also rate yourself on balance and body mass, and these factors will improve as you do strengthening, aerobic, and flexibility exercise.

KNOW THYSELF

Over the gates at Delphi are the words "Know thyself." This would be an apt inscription over every gym and workout facility in the world, for the core of success in gaining fitness is knowing yourself. Athletes have a very good sense of their goals: They want to run a 10k, they yearn for toned arms or abs, they want to lower their cholesterol. They know with absolute certainty where they are going. One problem: They don't know where they are. Most fitness-seekers eagerly slip into their shoes and head out into a training program essentially blind to their body's current condition and to their needs. Sadly, it's often an algorithm for aggravation.

Jeff, 32, came to us for testing. Jeff is big, 6'2", and very strong. He has lifted weights since college. "I'm pretty fit," he says. "I lift four times a week."

We administered our standard treadmill test, among others, and discovered that Jeff couldn't walk uphill; his aerobic fitness was as poor as someone who hadn't left the comfort of his couch for ten years. Jeff was stunned. To him, big biceps have always spelled fitness. Strong muscles *are* a part of fitness, but they aren't all of it.

Vanessa, 38, was a committed and disciplined runner. She made time to run every day and had a high level of cardiovascular fitness. Because she enjoyed running so much, she had never explored lifting weights, or doing any muscular strengthening or flexibility exercise such as Pilates or yoga. Not so surprisingly, she had very poor muscular and core strength, and recurrent back pain.

Melinda, too, looked very fit because she raced bikes on weekends. Recently, however, a routine scan at her doctor's office revealed she had osteopenia, a condition in which bone mineral density is lower than normal, though not low enough to be osteoporosis.

We believe it is crucial that you test yourself because, as these examples show, a person's perception of her fitness level is not always accurate. People may think they are very fit simply because they belong to a club or gym, while others might believe they are *not* fit even though their daily life or job includes lots of movement and activity. Some super-strong men with big upper bodies can easily bench-press two hundred pounds, but when tested, they prove to have poor flexibility and get winded easily. A carpenter or a grocery clerk who thinks he is completely unfit may test fairly high. Some cyclists with fantastic aerobic conditioning have poor flexibility and cannot lift forty pounds. For these reasons, testing in each area is the only objective means of determining your starting point.

ALTERNATE HARD AND EASY DAYS IN EACH AREA OF FITNESS

After you have established your starting point, you will calendar twelve weeks of aerobic exercise sessions at the precise length and intensity we advise. If you have a low aerobic score, you will dedicate more of your time to aerobic activities to give yourself a broad aerobic base; if (or, later, when) you merit a higher score, you will be instructed to focus most of your time working on your power, speed, and endurance. Your program evolves as you evolve, through the adjustments, retesting, and reevaluations we will give you.

We also furnish specific instructions on which days to skip a workout to allow your aerobic system to rest, and which days to go hardest, all with the goal of maximizing improvement. (More on this in Chapter 6, "Better Progress.") Then we serve up an array of aerobic exercise activities from which you can choose. You can walk, run, climb stairs, do aerobic circuit training, take a spin class, dance, train on an elliptical or StairMaster machine, or do one of a wide range of other activities. Almost all of the activities we recommend also help with proprioception, a component of balance. (More on that later.)

We also provide some guidance on selecting activities best suited to those who have some of the major risk factors. For example, if you have a high Body Mass Index, you will choose from a list that includes walking, swimming, or moderate cycling rather than running or taking a high-intensity step class. If you have another specific concern or limitation, we may offer you activities that will be easy on that specific part of your body, such as swimming, cycling, walking, Nordic skiing, in-line skating, or recumbent bicycling. Walking or running on grass, sand, trails, or a treadmill may be better for others. An elliptical trainer is even easier on the knees than a treadmill. Can't do weight-bearing activity? You can swim.

If you have no risk factors and are good to go, the exercise world is your banquet; you can choose any activity that uses large muscles in a rhythmic way. Our hope is that you try a number of different activities, with your family and friends, and find something—or several things—you will enjoy doing for the rest of your life.

What drew me to activity as a child was family involvement. I started skating at age two. My grandparents lived on a lake, so in cold weather I always had a sheet of ice. I joined a skating club at eight, raced nationally, and at fourteen started dreaming about the Olympics.

My grandfather was a hockey coach and part of the physical education department at the University of Wisconsin. Sports was always a part of our family activity. Some families play music, some dance; we did sports—*playing* sports, not observing. I believe that trying a number of different sports exposes you to the different nuances, the different pleasures of sports, and it's a great way to find something you can continue for the rest of your life.

—Eric

After we have designed your aerobic program, we will then go through the same steps to design your muscular strengthening package. Ditto for your flexibility regimen. As you weave together these three types of exercise, your balance and body composition will simultaneously profit from your efforts. In addition we recommend flexibility training, along with two sets of specific stretching exercises. These are based on the plans our patients receive; we will indicate the right one for you, based on your flexibility score, and instruct you on how to use it.

As we mentioned, there are four exercise modalities that your body needs regularly: aerobic conditioning, strengthening, flexibility, and balance and coordination. In short, we will give you all the tools necessary to assemble, manage, and understand your fitness program in all of these areas.

TREAT EXERCISE LIKE THE POWERFUL DRUG THAT IT IS

Hard, any, or random exercise, or simply more exercise is not guaranteed to make you better. To make the greatest use of the shortest amount of time to achieve fitness, you've got to take your exercise prescriptively—at the right time, in the right amount, at the right intensity, and for the right duration. And no more.

High intensity is not necessary; pain is not part of the ideal fitness program. In fact, high-intensity exercise often works against people, causing fatigue, burnout, even injuries. For people with hypertension, coronary artery disease, and other risk factors, high-intensity exercise also creates higher risk. So we always advance the lowest intensity necessary for people to improve. The good news for people who are already fit is that the ideal fitness program will focus your time and energy on the areas where you have weaknesses, so you, too, can experience great improvement.

Our plan dedicates the minimum number of hours doing the correct exercise at the lowest intensity necessary for you to experience fitness. It may require as little as four to six hours per week. That may seem like a lot, but how much time per day do you dedicate to eating? resting? working? What's one hour a day for something that will improve your life as profoundly as fitness?

EXERCISE IS LIKE A PRESCRIPTION DRUG

If you walk five days a week for a half hour a day, you will reduce your cholesterol, control your weight, and improve multiple systems within your body, according to the American College of Sports Medicine. The objective with this kind of exercise is to get healthier. And it works. As Sampath Parthasarathy, Ph.D., acclaimed biomedical researcher at Emory University, wrote in the *Journal of the American Heart Association*, "Regular exercise acts like a vaccine on the immune system."

Exercise is powerful medicine. It's not just something the U.S. surgeon general dreamed up to get you out of the house. There are definite, provable biological effects of exercise. We have watched how exercise *makes people healthier, often in profound ways*. We have also seen how twisting the knobs of exercise for our athletes—already very healthy people—could dial in progressively better fitness. We realized that when people suffer from disease, they may need medication. And they may need to kick-start their body's powerful ability to improve through exercise. We watched the studies pile up—multiple studies in many branches of medicine—detailing how specific forms of exercise trump just about anything else a person can do to improve her overall health, quality of life, and longevity.

Exercise, particularly aerobic exercise, acts as a drug. If you need to, say, lower your blood pressure, reduce your resting heart rate, or lower your risk of cardiac arrhythmia, there are prescription medications you can take—and you can take up an aerobic activity such as walking. Most people would experience similar benefits without the side effects of medication. Statins (medications popular for lowering cholesterol and reducing the risk of heart attack and stroke), for example, carry potential side effects involving your liver and muscles. Regular exercise does not.

- Aerobic exercise also acts like a beta-blocker, a medication often prescribed to people with high blood pressure. However, pharmaceutical beta-blockers can reduce physical performance and erectile function, which exercise doesn't do.
- Exercise increases your muscles' sensitivity to insulin. If you exercise regularly, your body needs to release less insulin. Our patients who are insulin-dependent diabetics discover that they require less insulin when they exercise. If someone is genetically disposed to develop diabetes by age forty-five and he exercises regularly, he may not develop it until age sixty, if at all.
- Aerobic exercise mirrors the effect of drugs that increase your HDL (good) cholesterol. A number of people with high cholesterol (or who currently take cholesterol-lowering medication for moderately but not severely elevated cholesterol) could do as well with a good exercise program and diet.
- Exercise performs the same function as diet pills in a weight-loss program.
- Lifting weights increases muscle mass and bone density, an effect similar to that of taking anabolic steroids or drugs for osteoporosis.

These are definite biological effects of exercise that you can measure. In fact, many modern drugs are designed to parrot the effects of aerobic exercise in order to treat diseases related to inactivity, including:

- coronary artery disease (heart attacks)
- cerebrovascular disease (stroke)
- hypertension, diabetes, excess weight, obesity, high cholesterol
- musculoskeletal diseases (decreased muscular strength, bone density, joint ROM/degenerative arthritis)
- cancer: colon, breast, prostate
- COPD (lung disease)
- depression and mood disorders

As we have slowed our level of movement and activity as a culture, these diseases have become frighteningly commonplace. Lack of exercise may be slowly crushing us as we age. And unlike a broken arm or sore throat, with most of these diseases the damage is done long before symptoms grab our attention. All of these diseases *can* be treated with drugs, but what those drugs accomplish is often biologically reproducible by exercise.

People who become active discover that they can reduce or eventually eliminate medications; many who are at risk for a disease often find they can remain disease- and drug-free if they are active. Ultimately, patients do better with exercise. And if you are already fit, this news should only bolster your resolve to stay that way.

If you already have been diagnosed with coronary artery disease, severely elevated cholesterol, diabetes, asthma, high blood pressure, or other chronic conditions, continue to take all medications prescribed by your doctor. However, after you have been taking the additional prescription of exercise for a while, your doctor may discover you can reduce your medication.

BETTER YEARS AND MORE YEARS

A body that's active may also be around longer. A Harvard Medical School study of more than forty thousand adults that began in 1960 found that exercise along with quitting smoking can add almost four years to your life, *even if you start at middle age or beyond.* Among those in the study who were seventy-five to eighty-four years old, exercising and quitting smoking added almost two years to their lives. The study also pointed out that those who enjoyed the benefits of a longer life were not necessarily signing up for triathlons, or even spin classes or weight lifting; less arduous activity did the trick as well. People can benefit with just thirty minutes a day of brisk walking, golf, tennis, gardening, or swimming. And it doesn't have to be continuous—you can break a thirty-minute session into two fifteen-minute parts. What's important is the total amount of energy expended.

We've already mentioned that many factors related to your health are genetic 10 to 25 percent. The remaining 75 to 90 percent is influenced by how you live. Certain cancers, for example, are caused primarily by environmental factors and lifestyle practices. Researchers started to realize this when people with low cancer rates migrating to places with high cancer rates began to show higher rates of cancer after adopting the lifestyle of the new area.

And as you get older, what you do on a daily basis has even more clout, according to the MacArthur Foundation Study of Aging in America. "If I had known I would live this long, I would've taken better care of myself" could not be more apt. Even low levels of exercise can pack a wallop when it comes to longevity, regardless of genetics. You have a tremendous amount of control over how you feel and how long you live. And most of that comes down to how much exercise you give your body. The lifestyle decisions you make every day yield how you will look, feel, move, and even think at forty or eighty. A nineteen-year study performed by the University of Helsinki, Finland, and published in the *Journal of the American Medical Association* ascertained that among fifteen thousand same-sex twins where one was physically active (defined as exercising as little as six times per month, for thirty minutes per session, at the intensity of vigorous walking) and the other twin was sedentary, the twin who exercised had a *55 percent lower risk of death* than the sibling who did not exercise.

FUEL YOUR BODY WITH THE RIGHT FUEL AND FLUIDS

When Kyle came into our clinic for the first time, he weighed more than three hundred pounds. He had come in for counseling on how to lose weight. His insurance required him to lose thirty pounds to be eligible for gastric bypass surgery, or stomach stapling, which would help him lose the majority of his unwanted weight.

The initial exam required that we record numerous body measurements, but it was difficult to find his knee, his neck, and his waist for all of the folds. He was thirty years old.

When we handed him an exercise plan, he looked shocked. But he had to start moving. Kyle's exercise prescription included low-impact aerobic activities (aquaerobics, swimming, and recumbent bike), some strengthening exercises organized in circuit training, and some Pilates exercises.

He started out reluctantly but kept his aspirations foremost, and in time he started seeing success. Over time, small successes added up to great success. In less than a year, Kyle lost *eighty pounds*. Kyle was so motivated by this that he came to us again, this time to get information on riding a bike. At first we prescribed only flat rides on a mountain bike with slick tires.

Kyle showed up in our office a year later and we hardly recognized him. He came in dressed like a Tour de France rider and rolling a nice road bike, ready for some testing to track his performance. His weight was down to 180 pounds.

Kyle never got bypass surgery. Instead, he joined a bike club and now he rides centuries, one hundred miles in a day.

Regular exercise goes hand in hand with weight loss. The extra weight anyone carries is stored fuel that his or her body needs to burn, simple as that.

Some programs promote the idea that you lose weight simply because you burn a certain number of calories while you're exercising. But there's more to the dynamic exercise and weight-loss duo than that. You also continue to burn calories *after* you exercise. The longer and harder you exercise, the longer your body will continue to burn calories. This can last for hours; for a Tour de France rider, it can last overnight. You may no longer be moving, but internally your chemical processes and enzymatic activity are still churning away. We call this exercise afterburn.

Exercise afterburn requires calories above and beyond what you've already burned, in order for your body to return itself to its pre-exercise state.

These calories are used to:

- replenish your glycogen stores (the way you store fuel in your muscles and liver)
- repair the wear and tear on your muscles caused by exercise (and these patch kits are made up of protein, which is costly in terms of calories)
- produce the hormones exercise induces (which also require protein)

To accomplish these tasks requires calories, and you get more bang for your bike ride with the right nutrients, and we'll show you which to give the highest priority.

Getting in Touch with Your Inner Tube

We likewise advance general instructions for selecting and using gear such as shoes, bikes, and gym equipment, but also for getting in touch with your own body and the signals it sends you as you exercise and may suffer injury. Selecting gear and doing the most popular activities safely is, of course, key to a lifelong exercise habit. And starting the habit of keeping an exercise diary will help you track your progress and learn the nuances of your changing health and body. If a problem should arise, you'll know how to assess your problem, pinpoint when it started, rate its severity, and communicate that problem to a health professional when necessary.

At this point, you will have in hand an exercise blueprint you will follow for the next twelve weeks. It will include the ideal frequency, intensity, duration, and type of aerobic, strengthening, and/or flexibility activity you need to do as you head out to exercise every day—your exercise "prescription," if you will. You will need to follow it carefully for reasons that will become clear. But we ask that you write your program ahead on your calendar only one week at a time, or in pencil, because success in fitness often depends upon going with the flow. Realistically, adjustments may need to be made due to illness, injury, scheduling conflicts, work, and other stressors, and you want to allow room for those adjustments. In the meantime, you will be armed with a highly personalized twelve-week fitness program—and you will understand what you're doing to your body, why you need to do it, and why it will work for you.

TRAIN YOUR BRAIN

We have been working with athletes—from top competitors who train for hours every day, to businesspeople and new parents with little time to train—and still almost every one comes to us at some point with the same questions:

"I start a workout program, but I never get better. Why?"

"I was once very fit, but since surgery/childbirth/my new job/retiring/ turning forty or fifty or sixty or seventy, I have lost it. How do I get back on track?"

"My friend does a certain workout at the gym. Can I just copy hers?"

"I work out like crazy, but I never lose weight. What am I doing wrong?"

"I make plans to be more active, but they never seem to materialize. How can I get started?"

"I know everything about training, but, um, what should I do?"

For most fitness-seekers, a lack of answers leads to disinterest, frustration, and failure. As physicians, we have observed that the road to fitness success is paved with scientific facts. Maybe you know about getting fit—you have read all of the books and magazines, you love exercise but never seem to achieve your goals. Or perhaps you are out of shape. Rest assured, neither one is a final diagnosis. A physician can make very few absolute guarantees, but there is one we make with confidence: You can get better, no matter your age or current condition. Our experience is that even knowledgeable athletes have never been exposed to the basic science of fitness, but once we arm them with nothing more than knowledge, many people start improving their fitness and health *today*.

Why Aerobic Exercise?

We give aerobic activity the highest priority. If you have time in your week for just one thing, make it aerobic. Why? The disease processes that are slowed or halted via aerobic exercise are much more likely to be fatal than those improved by strength training or by exercises that work flexibility and balance and coordination.

Aerobic activities include biking, jumping rope, running, swimming, step or water aerobics, Spinning, dancing (aerobic, swing, jazz, hula, flamenco), riding a stationary bike, Jazzercise, Frisbee, golf (walking the course), basketball, soccer, climbing stairs, and walking at a brisk pace (at a mall, around a track, or on a treadmill). But activity does not have to be done at a gym to modify your body and health. Actively playing with children, scrubbing the floor, mowing the lawn, raking leaves, and washing or waxing a car counts as well. What matters is not the exercise modality but the energy you expend. The important thing is to choose activities you can pursue for a lifetime.

Your ancestors certainly weren't going to the gym or taking Spin classes. They derived their physical fitness from sheer labor. Besides making sports part of your family culture, there are also the activities of daily life that you can embrace with greater gusto to get an aerobic workout. The following list from the Centers of Disease Control includes chores along with sports, to give you a sense of the comparative durations necessary to make them effective aerobic activities.

- Washing and waxing a car for 45–60 minutes
- Washing windows or floors for 45–60 minutes
- Playing volleyball for 45 minutes
- Playing touch football for 30–45 minutes
- Gardening for 30–45 minutes
- Wheeling yourself in a wheelchair for 30–40 minutes
- Walking 1¾ miles in 35 minutes (20 min./mile)
- Shooting baskets for 30 minutes
- Bicycling 5 miles in 30 minutes
- Dancing fast (social) for 30 minutes
- Pushing a stroller 1½ miles in 30 minutes
- Raking leaves for 30 minutes
- Walking 2 miles in 30 minutes (15 min./mile)
- Doing water aerobics for 30 minutes
- Swimming laps for 20 minutes
- Playing wheelchair basketball for 20 minutes
- Playing a game of basketball for 15–20 minutes
- Bicycling 4 miles in 15 minutes
- Jumping rope for 15 minutes
- Running 1½ miles in 15 minutes (10 min./mile)
- Shoveling snow for 15 minutes
- Stair climbing for 15 minutes

Becoming aerobically fit is not just a matter of teaching your muscles to do more work; it's a matter of teaching your body how to better utilize energy, from your lungs and heart down to the energy factories in your very cells. When you are aerobically active on a regular basis (almost daily), your lungs learn to breathe more effectively and your heart pumps more blood. Your blood thins, which keeps it flowing at a better clip; your blood vessels learn to move blood more effectively, and your arteries remain cleaner. You lower your cholesterol and blood pressure. Your blood itself carries more oxygen per minute. All of these reinforcements spell a major triumph in the trench warfare your body wages just performing normal, basic functions 24/7. This takes a load off your heart and your circulatory system, specifically, which means you are less likely to develop cardiac problems, such as coronary disease or congestive heart failure. Aerobic exercise also keeps your weight down and you gain energy. The longer you include exercise in your life, the longer lasting the improvements to the function of your heart and lungs will be. The measurement we use to assess this improvement is called VO2max.

Your VO2max represents how well your heart, lungs, and blood are delivering oxygen to your working muscles. To perform any sustained physical activity, you need to recharge the energy in your muscles by combining oxygen with fat and sugar. In this process, oxygen availability is the limiting factor for high-intensity efforts. How well your system transports oxygen (how well your heart, your lungs, your blood, and your muscles work together to get oxygen from the environment to the muscle fibers in order to produce energy) relates directly to the overall health and fitness of your cardiorespiratory system.

Meanwhile, all of your cells learn how to use energy more efficiently. And that includes the cells in your brain, which means you are more alert and better able to concentrate and for longer periods. Because regular exercise delivers more oxygen to your cells, every cell has better transport of food and waste; each cell functions better and lives longer. As you huff and puff your way through a workout, your mitochondria (the little energy plants within your cells) also increase in number and density, and each mitochondrion gets bigger and more active. This may be why studies show that you lose less function with aging if you exercise.

The foundation of your health is not just lack of disease; it's how optimally your body operates. How magnificently you perform is determined at the most basic level by the function of every cell in your body. Poor cellular function is the basis of many diseases, from cancers to heart disease. Cellular problems lead to organ and system malfunctions and failures. Impaired cellular and organ function is also how we measure aging and lack of fitness. Exercise pumps more blood—and essentially more oxygen-rich blood—to every one of those cells. With aerobic exercise, each cell is strengthened. When each cell is healthier, it functions better and is better able to stave off disease. With every cell running on all cylinders, every organ in your body operates at peak level. Improved cellular and organ action physiologically mirrors that of a younger person. In other words, your body enjoys vastly better overall health.

Why Strength Training?

The second most significant modality in your exercise routine is strength training. A longitudinal test of 993 men, published in the *Journal of Applied*

Physiology, shows that poor muscle strength is associated with a higher rate of mortality. Subjects' strength proved more important than traditional risk factors such as family history of heart disease, diabetes, and other diseases. In another study, researchers used the strength of the biceps, specifically the ability to bend the elbow, as the indication of the level of fitness. Why? If you have good muscle strength, most likely you also have a good cardiovascular system because you have been doing something to keep those muscles strong. People who lose strength are at higher risk for disease. If you have a chronic health problem, in all likelihood you are not very strong.

Strength training can be performed using machines, free weights, or your body weight (via push-ups, sit-ups, squats, wall push-ups, abdominal crunches, biceps curls, and overhead presses), and with activities including Pilates, yoga, plyometrics, and rock and stair climbing. You can also build strength by exercising with resistance bands, surgical tubing, or medicine or stability balls. (Part Two contains instructions for some exercises and routines. However, we cannot possibly supply specific routines for each sport or activity. To delve more deeply into specific sports, we suggest you seek expert advice in that sport.)

As noted above, the CDC (as well as other expert agencies) also note that good and effective strength-training activities include such household tasks as climbing ladders, and lifting and carrying groceries, boxes, garbage, buckets, gardening items, and, of course, children.

Strength training is vital for you in part because it is the most motivating exercise modality. When you start muscular strengthening, you see improvement quickly. You feel the benefits after just a few weeks and can see as much as a 20 percent improvement in just three months. Your muscles get bigger and better defined. Your body looks firmer and has better tone. Because lifting weights works your core (back and abdomen), you also lose abdominal fat, which has been shown to lower your risk for heart disease. As you gain muscular health, you increase your muscular endurance, which means you can perform regular daily activities longer before you tire, and you recover more quickly after doing them.

Strength-training exercise can also improve your skeleton, by bumping up your bone density. Your muscles use your bones as levers or pulleys. When you lift a weight with your arm, for example, the muscles contract to lever the bones in your arm upward. This leverage exerts force on the bone. This force stimulates the production of denser bone to reinforce those areas and—voilà!—better bone density. Research shows that professional weight lifters, for example, have much denser leg and spinal bones than their non-weight-lifting counterparts. The upshot is: Your bones that bear weight will grow denser. Denser bones suffer fewer and less severe musculoskeletal injuries. That can be very meaningful over a lifetime because the longer you go without these injuries, the longer you will be able to do the things you enjoy, and the less limited your existence will be. After all, research shows that beyond age thirty, you lose muscle mass every year. Over the long haul, you want to stay strong enough to get in and out of chairs, cars, and the bathtub unassisted, and to stay on your feet once you get there. All of this requires strength training today.

Strength training also puts the pedal to metal on your weight loss, because with it you gain muscle mass, and—pound for pound—maintaining muscle utilizes more calories than fat.

When I worked as a young family physician in Italy, on Lake Como, I was a member of a rowing club. The club competed in the annual Venice Marathon: six hundred rowing boats, forty-two kilometers. We had an eight-man boat, and *three of the men were over sixty-five, and one was over seventy.* Some of them were former national or world champion rowers. Three others were in their forties and fifties and very strong. At thirty-eight, I was the youngest on the team. Our club finished in the top ten several years in a row, competing against clubs that included people of all ages.

I had admired these older men since I was a kid; they were super fit, always. Later, as their family physician, I came to appreciate what good shape they were in physiologically: Each one's body functioned better than that of a thirty-year-old. They remained muscular, not soft or fat. These rowers also enjoyed the lifestyle of young men, filled with vitality, swimming in the lake, riding their bikes to the club, and living independently and medication-free.

I believe that their medicine was to go rowing every day.

—Max

Why Flexibility Exercise?

The importance of flexibility in your life cannot be overstated. Without it, your ability to do either of the first two exercise modalities—aerobics or strength building—is slowly eroded as you age, as is your ability to perform or enjoy normal daily activities. Diminished flexibility is not a given as you grow older. We have worked with dancers and yoga practitioners in their seventies who can fold themselves in half like a book, much like young adults. You can improve your flexibility through such activities as gymnastics, dancing, climbing, yoga, skipping rope, stretching, Pilates, ballet, water workouts, Tai Chi and other martial arts, range of motion activities, and exercise with elastic tubing or a balance ball.

Think of your muscles as dough. Passive stretching increases your muscle temperature, and as the muscle gets warmer, the "viscosity" of the muscle gets lower; the muscle becomes more fluid and longer, which gives you greater range of motion. Exercise requires muscles to stretch and contract. Stretching before you begin allows more optimal exercise, with less trauma to your muscles. Movement that increases your flexibility also bathes your joints in a lubricant called synovial fluid, which keeps them healthy.

Your muscles naturally stiffen as the years pile up. As you age, your muscle cells die and are replaced. When you do not engage in activities to increase your flexibility, your muscles lose collagen along with contractile fibers, which are strong and flexible, and these are replaced with fibrotic cells, which are less elastic and stiffer, akin to scar tissue. As that happens, you lose strength and flexibility. However, if you perform flexibility exercises, your dying muscle cells are instead replaced with flexible, contractile fibers, and go on to contract another day. (The muscle fibers in your heart can also stiffen with age but remain flexible with exercise.)

The aerobic and strength-training exercise you'll be doing will also cause your muscles to contract. Stretching exercises bring muscles back to their proper length. As you will see, it's better to stretch after warming up, which sets in motion greater blood flow to your extremities as well. The adrenaline you naturally release when you are under stress also causes muscles to contract and tighten; stretching loosens their grip and relieves tension. Likewise, muscles shorten with lack of use, and joints freeze up. This can cause a hunched or curled posture and limbs. The process can be speeded up by disease but also by lack of movement. If you have ever spent time in a cast, you've probably experienced a frozen joint. Not moving your joints regularly in their full range of motion causes the sleeve over your joints to shrink down to the smallest size possible for the range within which you are using the joint. If you move your joints only thirty degrees, after five years your joints will *be able* to move only thirty degrees. Without exercise that takes your joints through their full range of motion, you may eventually have difficulty taking off your shirt or shoes, combing your hair, putting on a necklace, or picking up objects from the floor. These are commonly the first symptoms people notice. People with sedentary jobs or lifestyles are most vulnerable. Core muscles—your trunk and pelvis—are not immune either. A flexibility routine that strengthens your core muscles will furnish the brace of support needed to help you prevent poor posture, lower back pain, and muscle injuries such as hernias.

A full range of motion does not just improve your chances of performing a layup in basketball or getting that bowl onto the top shelf. According to the Mayo Health Clinic, flexibility activities enhance your coordination as well, which may keep you on your feet far longer than your counterparts who don't exercise. A full range of motion means you're more likely to be able to put out a hand or a foot to catch yourself if you start to fall, thus avoiding a possible life-threatening injury. A full range of motion also translates to remaining light on your feet and never starting to fall to begin with. The investment might be fifteen minutes a day of flexibility exercise now, but the long-term benefit may be basic independence (the ability to dress, open a bottle, or bathe without help) at a later age. Movement, reach, and the ability to bend can increase dramatically—and inflexibility is delayed—when you stretch regularly.

Why Balance and Coordination?

Why work on balance? you ask. After all, you aren't planning on walking a tightrope anytime soon.

Down the road, when you're in your sixties or eighties, just walking across the room may feel as if you're walking a tightrope if you haven't worked on balance. Without coordination and strength, you are less likely to regain your balance if you take a misstep. And one of the top challenges after sixty-five concerns a lack of balance: falls. These too often result in hip fractures, which for many are as life threatening as walking a tightrope. Of the 250,000 people who fracture a hip every year, 20 percent die, according to the National Institute of Arthritis and Musculoskeletal and Skin Diseases. Some of those who survive may face life in a nursing home, unable to walk, watching the world through a TV set.

You work on balance and coordination anytime you do aerobic, strengthening, or flexibility activities, but the movement that best improves balance and coordination is that which tests your equilibrium: all the way from walking on uneven surfaces such as trails or rocks to standing on cushions or new devices designed to exercise balance. Balance and coordination are refined by martial arts, gymnastics, water aerobics, yoga, Pilates, Tai Chi, bicycling, dance, fishing, rowing, skiing or snowboarding, riding a scooter, mountain biking, cyclocross, surfing, kickboxing, climbing, and—one of Eric's favorites—skating.

Exercise that enhances your body's coordination and sense of balance is vital, because as you age your movements naturally grow slower and more imprecise. You need to compensate for normal advancing muscle weakness with better balance when walking down stairs or rising from a chair. Unable to rise from a chair without using your arms? This is a sign that your balance, and the muscles required to maintain balance, need work.

From our observations, it seems that people with intellectual jobs— teachers, lawyers, and, well, doctors—lose agility more quickly than those who are employed using their elbow grease, doing manual labor. The reason? The latter are practicing their balancing act five days a week, eight hours a day. And they retain smoother movement into old age.

Don't want to change careers? Your other option is exercise. Exercise of all kinds hones not only your body but also your body's communications with its control tower, your brain. It does this through what's called proprioception. Proprioception is your inner sense of the position of your body parts, where they are in relation to one another and with respect to the space around you. Close your eyes and check in with your body parts: Where are your feet? Are they flat on the floor or splayed out in front of you? How about your hands? How do you know without looking? That's proprioception at work. When you have a high degree of proprioception, you know without looking, for example, the exact location and position of your arms, and the precise angle of your body with respect to the ground. Proprioception profits as you exercise, and your balance and your ability to avoid falls profit with it. If you know the location of your feet and arms, for example, and you are on good speaking terms with them, when you start to fall you will stick one of them out in a flash, in time to stop the fall.

Researchers participating in the Study of Osteoporotic Fractures, funded by the National Institutes of Health (NIH), followed more than 9,500 older women with numerous risk factors for hip fracture over four years. They discovered that subjects cut their risk of hip fracture *by one-third* just by walking regularly for exercise. The farther the women walked, the lower their risk. Researchers also learned that women decreased their risk of hip fracture if they did no walking but just spent four hours or more per day *on their feet.*

Regular balance and coordination activities sharpen your wiring and speed up the transmission of signals from your toes to your brain and back again. This keeps your movements smooth and precise with respect to your environment. Exercise also keeps your inner ear in tune, another factor that influences balance. Contrary to what many people believe, balance and coordination are trainable, and those who adopt activities requiring them can retain peak coordination.

Exercise Is Not Just for Jocks

There is also a misperception that fitness belongs to a certain type of person, that exercise is just for jocks. But fitness is in fact for *everyone.* You are exquisitely designed for movement. The human body and brain originally developed, in fact, to serve movement.

Our evolution as a species, like that of other creatures, started with the need to move. Early brains had to juggle a vast number of signals coming in from the environment (the steepness of the path, the location of a branch) and from the body itself (the position of the foot, the level of fatigue). This brain then had to simultaneously fire out signals to the muscles in order for them to move within that set of circumstances. It was the ultimate in multitasking. Over time, as the human brain improved its ability to coordinate muscle contractions in response to stimuli, we also learned how to use the brain to assess and respond to dangers, to analyze situations in a conscious way, and to memorize experiences. Most of your brain is dedicated to coordinating the actions of your muscles. Your brain causes your muscles to contract, which shortens the distance between your bones, and you move. The more you move, the more you learn, taking in billions of bits of information about the pressure on your joints, the tension in your muscles.

Scientists also hypothesize that our incredible ability to adapt—to live in such varied climates, to eat such diverse foods—has its origin in our ability to move.

Researchers now believe that the ability of muscle to contract in a supervised way is what developed our brain into the incredible machine it is today. It is no wonder that the creatures with the most sophisticated forms of movement have the largest, most advanced brains.

Many of the functions we perform (breathing, heartbeat, balance) are still organized by a portion of our brain that operates below our awareness, while the superior part of our brain—the cortex—allows us to consciously control movement (I want to walk over there; I want to go quickly). Activity has forced the human brain to grow in order to be ready for whatever challenges future movement might present.

Movement makes up a fundamental component of our evolution and of life. Like the main beam that holds up a house, how much you move affects your strength, your power, your balance, how you look, how you think, how well you withstand the high winds and rain showers of life, and how long you will stand. Movement is an essential biological requirement, as high on the human priority list as food, water, shelter, and air. People are often detached from their body's cries for exercise, however. You know that thirst signals your need for water, hunger expresses your need for food. When you are cold, you seek warmth, and a burning in your lungs makes you gasp for air. But when do you acknowledge that your body needs more movement? When your knees or your back ache? When you're tired all day but can't sleep at night? When all of your clothes seem to be shrinking? When your doctor announces that your cholesterol is much higher than last year, that your blood pressure or your Body Mass Index (weight to height ratio) is virtually off the charts?

You may not know it, but those numbers in your medical chart are your exercise report card. They are directly related to your *fitness level*. Good genes or an active job can protect you for a while, but eventually *every*one needs concentrated doses of several kinds of movement (aerobic, strength, flexibility, and balance and coordination) to remain fully functional. Over a lifetime, a lack of fitness evolves into a vicious cycle. Your metabolism slows when you don't exercise, so every activity becomes more difficult. In response you choose movements that are easier to do and demand less of your body, so you move less and burn fewer calories; you gain weight. The additional weight makes your joints sore. Sore joints cause you to reduce your range of motion; you don't want to reach high or bend low. When you reduce your range of motion, your joints become stiffer. Then all movement becomes difficult. So you avoid activity and gain more weight, which makes your joints even creakier, and so on . . . Whatever your genes or your exercise history, no one is immune to the ill effects of a lifestyle that doesn't include exercise.

Research has whipped the veil off the fact that when the human body lacks movement, it becomes more susceptible to disease, pain, weight gain, disturbed sleep cycles, unhealthy cravings, stiffness, loss of function, loss of balance, injury, weakness, and more. The World Health Organization reports that, of the world's adults—rural and urban, developing nation and developed—60 to 85 percent are inactive, and that 2 million deaths annually can be attributed to sedentary lifestyles, making inactivity one of the top ten causes of death in the world. In the United States alone, almost 850 people die every day due to inactivity—the third leading cause of death, right after heart disease and cancer. And those two diseases have been linked to inactivity as well.

However, even as you chalk up more birthdays, you maintain the ability to get better with exercise. Research shows that people sixty-five and better experience, on average, a 30 percent improvement in exercise efficiency, a parameter that refers to the amount of oxygen your body uses to perform a given task. Those in their twenties and thirties experienced a paltry 2 percent gain. Why? The subjects in their twenties were already efficient, while the ones in their sixties had a larger margin to gain—and gain they did.

Myriad facets of physical deterioration that you may think are inevitable signs of aging are actually symptoms of lack of use. A glimpse at a list of what deteriorates with age and a list of what improves with exercise, you will see that they are mirror images of one another:

Targets of Aging	Targets of Exercise
• Heart and arteries	• Heart and arteries
• Lungs	• Lungs
• Blood	• Blood
• Hormones	• Hormones
• Muscles	• Muscles
• Brain and nerves	• Brain and nerves
• Bones	• Bones

The Biology of Thought

It's important that you know these things because science also shows that there are biological consequences to the kinds of thoughts you entertain. If you know, for example, that many of the "problems of aging" can be halted, slowed, or reversed the more you use your body, you'll do better in your exercise program. If you acknowledge that, unlike a car, if you park yourself in a chair, you actually deteriorate faster, and that when you start putting on miles (on a treadmill, bicycle, sidewalk, trail, or dance floor), you will actually start purring like a well-oiled machine. And you *can* get better, no matter your age or starting level. True self-confidence comes not from convincing yourself that you can do something you cannot but from dealing positively with facts. The reality of your exercise challenges, and the benefits, can polish your self-confidence and fortify your motivation.

No matter your history, everyone can get moving and get better. Studies show that if you have never exercised, you will actually get better faster and with greater ease than those who are already active. Because the more unfit you are the more you have to gain, the greatest progress occurs at the low end of the scale. You will also show greater improvements in your risk factors and in your disease symptoms. Again, research has spotlighted that the biggest improvement in fitness and the most significant reduction in risk factors occur in the people with the lowest levels of fitness.

Look around you; become an observer of the human race. Notice the people who exercise regularly. They are often happier, more energetic, and less dependent on medication. Your sedentary friends of the same age are frequently tired, dealing with pain, taking lifelong medication, and coping with its cost and inherent side effects. The key is to recognize that lack of exercise is a disease that you have complete control over, a disease that you can start turning around as soon as you begin.

What are you doing today?

"A person will sometimes devote all his life to the development of one part of his body—the wishbone."

—Robert Frost

2

better goals

What is your goal?

Of all the people who start an organized exercise plan, 50 percent drop out within three months, defeated not by the exercise itself but by their goal. A meaningful and realistic purpose is critical to fitness success.

As we often say, there are no bad athletes, only bad goals.

In this chapter we will guide you in setting your objectives, then help you scrutinize them with great care. You will learn how to define your ambition, and to compare your aspirations to those we know come to fruition and those that don't. Then we will demonstrate how to reshape your desires, round them out, and buttress them to withstand your journey ahead.

> Throughout much of my life I have been considered a very goal-oriented person. Much of the success I have had has been the result of some dreaming, lots of planning, plenty of hard work and sweat, and a great deal of focus, dedication, and concentration.
>
> —Eric

The first step is the nucleus: your vision. Why do you want to get fit? Athletic aspirations are as numerous as the people who seek them. Perhaps you want to:

- have more energy
- look better
- improve your overall health and potential for longevity
- reduce genetic health risks
- have more fun
- lose weight
- gain a longer attention span
- attain a certain speed or performance level in your sport
- reduce cholesterol
- relieve stiffness and pain
- heal or avoid disease
- regain youthfulness
- live to see your grandchildren
- make up for poor treatment of your body in the past

Other apt objectives of exercise include those within the realm of activity itself:

- "I want to participate in a fund-raising walking/running/cycling/swimming event."
- "I want to get there faster than last time."
- "I want to finish in the top twenty."
- "I don't want to be left behind next summer on our biking vacation through the south of France."

All of these are noble and realistic fitness goals. Here's how to make them happen.

Set Goals by the Calendar, not the Clock

We are all eager to exercise—as long as we see results by tonight. Okay, maybe by the weekend. No one wants to wait to achieve their fitness objectives. We have been spoiled by slapping down a credit card, ordering things on the Internet, next-day delivery, and instant messaging for an immediate response. People who are accustomed to making things happen at the office or at home can be especially impatient. They want to see prompt changes in their fitness, too. People have seen it happen on reality TV; they think they can do a body makeover in two hours.

It takes a good three months to see results. So set your sights by the calendar, not the clock. Plan on achieving your aim by the end of the season or the end of the year, not by the weekend. Stick with it and be consistent, and improvement *is* going to happen. Fitness is not roulette: black or red, yes or no. And it's not like the lottery ("I've been taking a shot at it off and on all my life, but my number never seems to come up"), but more like taking a class or gardening ("Slowly but surely, I'm going to make this happen"). Moreover, the time it takes to achieve a goal is specific to you as an individual. It may look as if your best friend simply spun the wheel and hit the jackpot at the gym, while you have been on a losing streak. You need to understand that fitness follows a slow and winding but deliberate path, and if you stay on it you'll get there. If you keep this in mind, you will be less likely to stop and leave the path just as you were about to cross the threshold to visible improvement.

Set Reasonable Goals

As we say, if you're out of shape, it is not a final diagnosis. Even if you are out of shape in some ways, you might be in good shape in other ways. And scientifically, the more out of shape you are, the greater your chances for improvement. Why? Your body hungers for exercise and eagerly drinks up every possible benefit when you begin to exercise. But your potential to improve is not infinite. As an athlete achieves the majority of improvements that are possible within a certain sport, the potential for continued advancement is diminished. Those with the least potential for improvement are in fact the most elite athletes. This is because elite athletes have already pushed their body to the furthest reaches of what's humanly possible. However, in the arena of the elite where everyone is at the top end of the range, if an athlete is able to make even a 1 percent improvement, that may spell the difference between winning the race and coming in twelfth.

Mona was nearly fifty. She had run fifteen marathons. Her best time was five hours twenty-five minutes, her worst time five hours forty-five minutes. She very consistently ran twelve- to thirteen-minute miles. To complete past marathons, she had alternated running and walking, because she couldn't run the whole way.

Mona was a seasoned athlete. She had been exercising for a long time, so room for vast further improvement in the marathon was limited. But when I asked her about her aspirations, she said she wanted to break the four-hour mark, to qualify for the Boston Marathon.

For Mona to run a marathon in fewer than four hours would require trimming an hour and a half off her time. To do that, she would have to run nine-minute miles for the entire race—cutting off a quarter to a third of her time each mile. She had never maintained a nine-minute-mile pace, even when running much shorter races, such as 10ks.

"Why do you think you can achieve this?" I asked her.

"My yoga teacher told me that the only reason I have never broken the four-hour mark is because I have never really wanted to, that it's only a matter of mind-set," Mona replied. "If I really want to do it, I can do it."

"When is the marathon?" I asked.

"Three months from now," she replied.

"I would really like to meet your yoga instructor."

—Max

Mona was already doing well in running marathons—perhaps the best she could possibly do, and yet she was being encouraged to pursue a goal that was not reasonable. The truth is, there is much a person can achieve in fitness, but you can only do it *if you have the potential to do it.* If Mona, at 4'9" and ninety pounds, had decided she wanted to play for the NFL, I'm sure no one would have told her, "You have never played for the NFL simply because you never wanted to; if you really want to, you can do it." Many types of athletics require *invisible* gifts—physical qualities that are not apparent to the naked eye, attributes such as VO2max, trainability, rate of recovery, and so on. Mona's limitation might be any one of these, but because these gifts are not readily apparent, it's very easy for Mona and for others to fall prey to utterly unfounded proclamations, and that can set people up for disappointment.

Height is a requirement to play in the NBA, with very few exceptions. Basketball's height requirement is simple to accept and height is an easy gift to recognize. It's harder to accept that to run as well as your neighbor runs, or to respond as quickly to a weight program as your buddy does, you also must have the right gifts. Why? *Because you can't see those physi-*

cal characteristics. Perhaps these goals require the genes that grant a greater capacity to utilize oxygen or to build muscle, or any one of the many unseen qualities inside your cells, your muscle fibers, your organs, your blood, or your brain. In any given discipline, one of these concealed aptitudes might be as crucial to success as height is in basketball. Though enshrouded, these attributes are equally immutable. As they say, "You can't learn height."

Your goals in this program will play a significant role in your motivation, in your getting out the door every day. So it's crucial that your goals work in tandem with reality and that they do not inadvertently thwart your efforts by allowing your goals to instead hand you disappointments. You need to harness your motivation and experiencing success is a huge driving force. We often see this in top athletes. At the end of a grueling event in which everyone is on their last leg, something happens that gives them motivation. They are suddenly fresh and take off with renewed power.

This shows how dramatically your brain can modulate the way you feel fatigue and other sensations. This is why goals, novelty, and other factors are perhaps more important to fitness than the quality of your genes. You must enlist your brain in your quest for fitness, because it holds a great deal of power over exaggerating or minimizing the way you experience training.

So, yes, your mind-set is very important—it can give you the wings to overcome enormous hurdles, but to think it's *all* a matter of mind-set takes your attention off your true potential. No matter Mona's mind-set, for example, it is simply not possible for her to improve that significantly, that quickly, in a sport in which she has been training for years. When a person has already fully and expertly explored his limitations within a certain sport, even the best mind-set cannot propel him to achieve an objective that is an excessive reach beyond his upper limit, especially in an abbreviated amount of time. As physicians, we respect the psychological aspect of athletic success and focus on it with our athletes. We feel it's at least as important as the physiological aspects (see Chapter 10, "Better Motivation"). Your mind is, indeed, an incredible tool and you can use it to achieve your goals. Still, we all have physiological limitations, otherwise everyone could win the Tour de France. A hundred and eighty cyclists start the Tour de France every year, and every year only one wins. For one seven-year stint it was always the same guy (though the others were not that far behind). A big component of Lance Armstrong's success was certainly his incredible mental focus and his ability to really push himself, but attitude is not everything. He also possessed the necessary physical aptitude. As a self-coach, you will want to look at your goals and perhaps admit, "That goal isn't realistic for me. Maybe I can get there in three years; maybe I can never get there."

With Mona we modified her goal and decided to go for her personal best. To achieve this we sharpened all components of her performance: fitness, muscular endurance, skills, flexibility, nutrition, and mental focus. We carefully plotted her training and her tapering. The result? She ran a five-hour marathon. At age fifty, she was *twenty-five* minutes faster than she had ever been in the last fifteen years. That is success.

If you are willing to acknowledge the genetic limitations we all have without being discouraged, you will save yourself substantial time, energy, money, and grief. We have all been baited by unrealistic hopes; it's frustrating to work for months or years without achieving a heartfelt goal. But limited ability in one area doesn't mean you don't have potential. You will more effectively respond to exercise when you seek a fitness goal that is realistic and well suited to your invisible strengths.

Let's compare Eric and me. We are both physicians. Eric's father is a world-record holder for the 2,500-meter distance on the rowing machine at age seventy and won a national title as a masters cyclist in the time trial. Eric's sister won three world championships in two different sports. At age twenty-one, Eric won five gold medals as a speed skater in the Olympics. Dr. Heiden's five medals are in all distances, from sprinting to endurance. Then he became a cyclist, won the U.S. pro championship, and competed in the Tour of Italy and the Tour de France.

Me? I played soccer, did some skiing, rowing, and cycling. My father was an accomplished mountain climber and skier, but there aren't so many gold medals around our house.

You might conclude that Eric's genes are very different from mine. Objectively, you might also say that we should have different goals and expectations. You would be right.

Eric and I have a group bike ride we do together. Because he has the genetic ability to respond to exercise, he goes out the same number of times as everyone else in our group, but he gets much better than the rest of us very quickly.

"Hey, Eric," I tell him, "you are a freak."

Seriously, though, I know—we all know—that this is the nature of sport. Yes, Eric keeps leaving me behind. I just concentrate on bettering my own performance. There are other doctors we train with who are pretty much on my level, so when I want to compete I focus my efforts on trying to beat them. They are genuine competitors, not freaks.

—Max

How to Recognize Realistic Goals

If your purpose is to excel at a certain sport, ask yourself if realistically you may have already topped out. If you're just starting out at a new activity, be sure that your goal is compatible with your physical gifts, and if it is not move on to another, more reasonable goal. If, when just starting out in a sport, you discover steady improvements, you are very likely doing something at which you are gifted, and your upper limit is as yet unknown. Everyone is gifted at something, and in Part Two you will find out how to test yourself and discover your gifts.

After every skating season we would sit down with our coach and assess our previous season, then we would set realistic goals for the next year.

—Eric

Likewise, keep a clear head about what to expect regarding physical changes in your body and steer clear of harboring unrealistic weight goals. People are often discouraged in their quest for fitness not because they aren't achieving success but because they aren't achieving some *unrealistic ideal* of success.

Don't expect to lose fifty pounds in six weeks, or that your biceps will quickly bulk up, that fitness is like the dramatic "before" and "after" pictures in advertisements. Many people who have never been exposed to the science of fitness secretly believe the end point of fitness looks like the guy in the Bowflex ads. The endpoint of getting fit does *not* resemble the guy in the Bowflex ads. Even the guy who does the Bowflex ads doesn't resemble that guy, without the benefit of special lighting, makeup, airbrushing, and other effects. Maybe you won't lose fifty pounds; maybe you'll lose twenty, but it's better to lose twenty than none at all, or to keep steadily gaining weight. The real-world reward of fitness is a body that sings with a new level of health, vitality, and ability. It is being able to walk a certain distance effortlessly after a lifetime when that was impossible.

Make note of where you're starting. Once you begin to get fit, it's easy to forget where you started. People are quick to put out of their minds how slow or out of shape they once were. Or they say, "I was hoping I would get even faster or lose more weight," because their improvements were not as steep or as fast as they predicted. We have to remind them: "Remember when you came here last time you weren't able to jog three and a half miles an hour. Now you *walk* at that speed."

Along the way, remember that any improvement is improvement, and that fitness isn't always a dramatic achievement, as it seems in commercials for exercise machines. On the other hand, you may also lose *more* weight or see improvement *faster* than you expected—these factors rely upon your particular genetic predisposition. Everyone falls somewhere on the spectrum, but everyone is on the spectrum. Even a sedentary person who starts exercising two or three times a week will show progress after a month. We cannot remember a single patient who did the program who didn't improve. No matter your level, you will get better.

START WITH A MAIN GOAL

My main goal right now is to schedule three or four workouts a week. That's a big success—to get in six hours of exercise a week.

—Eric

Part of your main goal, or endpoint, should be something concrete that you want to achieve in the next season or year. Rather than choosing such nebulous goals as "feeling stronger," or "looking better in my clothes," target a certain amount of workouts or a certain frequency per week, participation in an event, achieving a certain distance or time, reaching a physical milestone (a specific weight or a *size* in clothing, for example), or being able to get through a Spinning class, say, without feeling like you're dying. If you do set performance goals, take the pressure off and set reasonable, limited goals, such as "I want to work up to bicycling 50/100/200 miles a week over the next six months," "I want to run a mile in nine minutes," "I want to be able to make it all the way through my workout without resting," or "I want to be in the top twenty at the end of a climb."

Incremental Goals

During the first three months you will also set smaller, more modest targets for yourself. Ideally, focus on behavioral objectives rather than performance goals for these. Allowing yourself to focus on behavioral goals in the short term offers a greater degree of guaranteed success. If you focus on winning the local 10k or a cycling criterium race in a month though you don't yet have a good training routine or haven't slowly ratcheted up your times, you need to work on the incremental improvements first. So set mini-goals to achieve along the way. Good aspirations also include walking for two minutes, running for one, walking for two minutes, running for three, working your way up; getting to the gym four times a week for a month; or sticking to a diet and fitness program for just this week, then this month, and so on. This will also help you create the fitness habit: *I want to go to the gym six days a week. I want to create a walking, running or cycling group with my friends. I want to bicycle to work every day. I want to climb the stairs every day at lunch for a month.* These are realistic behavioral aims because you have control over your behavior. The best incremental goals are those that ensure you're on track to achieving your main goal, for example:

"In the next two months I want to improve my time/weight/repetitions this much."

"I want to lose four pounds in the next month."

Keeping an eye on your subtle progress is motivating as you inch toward your major goal, this season and year by year. It's also an early warning system that alerts you to poor progress so that you can quickly make adjustments and not waste time on dead-end exercise. As you hit each mark, you can move to the next limited target.

My intermediate goal now is to keep my weight down. And my daily goal is to not get beaten up by my training partner, a friend and neighbor who starts pushing right out of the driveway.

—Eric

Again, neither your endpoint objective nor your incremental aims should be centered on someone else's performance, at least at the beginning and intermediate phases of your fitness experience. Tempting as it is to try to lose more weight than your neighbor or outperform your training buddy, scientifically there is no relevance to how someone else is doing; it's not an apt measure of your progress, and thus it makes a poor goal. This is about exercise, not competition. In focusing on comparisons rather than your individual progress, you may fail to notice things that aren't working, or you may not push yourself to new limits.

If you're a beginner, set incremental aims such as:

- pacing yourself during each phase of the workout so that you can finish the workout
- completing each workout *or*
- feeling good at the end of each workout

If you are intermediate, your mezzo-goals may be:

- to feel that a workout that was difficult in the beginning is now easy *or*
- to do what was undoable two months ago, and have it feel like a piece of cake

If you are advanced, a good interim wish would be to participate in a specific event.

As a beginning or intermediate athlete, you may find yourself getting discouraged because you do not have a sense of your limit. You may expend too much energy at the beginning of your workout and then hit a barrier later, because you don't quite know your body's limit yet. If you concentrate on pacing yourself, after a few workouts you'll know how far to go in the first five, ten, fifteen minutes, and throughout your workout so that you will be able to make it to the end. You will be able to ascertain your level of fatigue within the workout and gain control over it. Before long, you'll be able to say, "I can do it anytime I want—I own that workout."

To continue your development as an athlete, the logical progression is to feel you can put yourself with a group of people who exercise and feel good about it, to participate in an event. The event need not be competitive. It can be a local 5k or 10k walk, a fund-raising ride, or participating on a community team. Participating in an event is an important step in your physical improvement, a true leap to feeling even more comfortable with your own fitness. Too often people are afraid to participate when they are in poor physical condition, and they don't break that mind-set once they get fit. They still don't go along on a group hike, they still don't go to the swimming pool, they still don't take part in the company softball team or sign up for the fund-raiser. People invite them to participate and they continue to think, Everyone is so much better than I am. Instead, say yes, keep your thoughts positive, and focus on a realistic goal for yourself within the realm of participation.

The next step is to consider participating in a *competitive* event. Don't berate yourself with self-talk like "I don't have the numbers or ability to win this year." Instead, show yourself kindness, be gentle, and, again, focus on what is a realistic goal for you within this event. For example, "Right now I have great numbers, but they are not realistic for winning this event this year. Instead I'll focus on finishing in the top 25 percent for my age group." When you achieve that goal, your next aspiration might be to finish in the top 10 percent or to challenge yourself with longer distances.

The Starting Line

When you buy a car, you want to know everything about it: its engine size, its power capacity, its braking system, its fuel and maintenance needs, and so on. But what do you know about your body, the vehicle you use every moment of your life? Some people would just as soon not know. You do need to know, however, if you want to make upgrades through exercise. You may not have control over your genetics, but you do have complete control over your level of self-knowledge, and self-knowledge in this arena is very powerful. Collecting information about yourself and becoming aware of what is happening to your body are key instruments in your fitness tool kit.

When you decide to invest time in exercise, you need to establish your starting point—to know the size of your own engine, if you will. You can't get to Point B without first establishing Point A, your current condition. You will use physical tests to establish Point A. You can do your assessments at home or at a lab. We detail both in Part Two. The evaluations we recommend determine your aerobic status, your levels of muscular strength and flexibility, and your body composition. Once you have your physiologic profile, you will have your starting point on an objective scale and be able to use it to plot your progress as you train.

Objective testing is necessary to ascertain your starting point because you cannot gauge your ability by what you think of yourself. Ego and personality too often color the facts. Some athletes are very self-conscious and downplay themselves, for example. When asked about their abilities, they say, "I am just average." Yet with testing, it turns out that they have great potential. Other people say, "I am the next Lance Armstrong," but when tested, they reveal the scores of an average, sedentary subject. We know that training-induced improvements are complex and multifactorial (Was it how she slept? Or something else that's not being studied?). This makes training an inexact science. For this reason, you need to test yourself for your starting point and monitor your improvement over time.

The studies we depend on in designing programs are based on statistical averages. (Only those with any statistical weight—meaning sheer numbers of people studied—get published.) If they weren't, you wouldn't need to test. We could give everyone a list of exercises that are proven to be best in all groups, and everyone would get better. But you are an individual, and a particular technique may not be the best for you. When trying to improve *individuals*, custom-made plans make more sense, and that requires establishing who you are as an individual via testing. Moreover, many of the factors that determine your strengths and weaknesses are impossible for you to assess subjectively; you have to be measured scientifically. For this reason, testing can also bestow good news about your unknown strengths.

Testing Reveals Gifts

Christine Thorburg, herself a physician, came to us after having knee ligament reconstruction. She had been a cross-country runner in college and more recently had done some recreational cycling at age thirty, but that was about it.

Christine really enjoyed cycling, so she asked us to test her. When we saw her scores we realized that she had an exemplary physiology for cycling. She had never been tested before, had never known she would be good at the sport, and had never had a training program.

We said, "Too bad you didn't know about this before!"

We gave her a training program, and in one year she made the national cycling team. In two years she was the national champion and qualified for the Olympic time trials. In the Athens Olympics she came in fourth. And all this while continuing to work as a physician.

Like Christine, after testing, you will want to capitalize on what you *do* have. Exercise is great in that there are so many ways to be gifted: with flexibility, power, endurance, strength, coordination, balance, rhythm, mental focus, and so on. So discover the gifts that you have, and acknowledge that a lot of people wish they had your gifts, whatever they might be.

Have a Good Plan—and Use It

We may live in an age in which people *do* more, but we certainly don't plan more. Most people never plan when it comes to exercise. It's as if they want to sneak up on their workouts. They throw on their workout clothes and head out the door without a thought beyond how much time they have. Or they exercise year-round, year after year, the same way. It's as if they're afraid they will stop altogether if they think about it too much. And then they wonder why they don't lose the weight or feel better, why they have aches and pains, and why they're frustrated in meeting their goals. The result is that people do exercise that is of little benefit physiologically or could actually cause harm. That's why it's so important to have a good plan—and then stick to it.

> A lot of people spend time thinking about what they're doing. Every day when I go out, I know exactly what to do.
> —Levi Leipheimer
> Third Place, Tour de France 2007,
> and a client of Max and Eric

People come to our office and we help them put together a wonderful plan that virtually guarantees their goals will be met. An unbelievable number of them come back after six months with a long face and a shrug.

"I didn't improve as much as I expected to," they say.

So we ask, "How did you do with this part of the plan? How about that part?"

"Well, I didn't really follow the program because you know Tuesdays there's a group of friends I walk with who go at a different pace than the plan," they say. "And Thursdays I work late, and I swim weekends at the Y instead, so the plan we put together didn't really match my week."

And we think, So basically you're telling me that for six months you did exactly what you were doing before coming here. And you wonder why you didn't improve?

Once you have the will (your goal), you need to have a way (a program). In Part Two, once you have assessed yourself, we will instruct you on precisely what to do for your level of fitness. When you calendar your program, you will take into account the way your weeks normally unfold as you schedule your program.

This will be your program. The next big step is to follow the program.

Some people don't think they need to follow a plan for getting fit. Perhaps some people are in denial. Others might not have needed a plan when they were younger, and they don't realize how dramatically the body changes with age and how much more it requires targeted exercise to stimulate adaptations. Sometimes it's simply a matter of personality: They want to do it their own way. But often, the perceived problem is that a *doctor* conjured up a program, and they know the slow, meticulous march of science. They might think to themselves, I want something that works *fast*.

Speed is really at the heart of a lot of wasted energy and exercise effort: People want something fast. You need to be willing to till the soil for a season, however, if you want to eat the world's best tomatoes.

Exercise Is Like Marriage . . .

You need to remain faithful to your program, yes, but as in marriage, flexibility is also required. You may be compelled to tweak your program here and there during the long arc of time toward your goal. In Part Two we outline the precise adjustments you may need, given your responses to the exercise. But be aware that it may be difficult for you to remain flexible, especially if it requires going backward a bit. We were surprised at first by the number of coaches—even professional ones—who come to us for coaching. Why do they? Because it is difficult to coach yourself. But there is a way. You can coach yourself if you remain smart about it and follow a few guidelines. (By the way, if you are a coach and are reading this book to better teach your athletes, the guidelines for adjusting our program apply to coaching others as well.)

Adjustments represent the *art* of training (as opposed to the science). All training programs offer a vision and a design, with some mathematical rules, but basically these represent only the framework. Stick with the framework, but—to belabor the house metaphor—you'll need to open and close the windows depending on the weather. As a self-coach, you want to become the master of minor adjustments. No human being is the perfect average around which most science-based programs are designed, as we've said. You are not a machine; you are a genetically unique creature. Neither are your days identical. One day you might feel a certain type of fatigue or soreness. Another week you might miss a workout or two due to a work deadline. What do you do? Back off completely? Quit? Redouble your efforts? To be an effective self-coach, you need to know the basic principles of training and to understand what is going on with your body. A good training program or coach teaches you how to acknowledge and measure those factors to provide insight into yourself. Much of what you need to know is contained in this book. From there, you need to know that as an individual your responses will vary.

Whatever adjustments you need to carry out, remember that you will ultimately be rewarded. It's going to happen. If your goal is losing weight, if you do more and don't eat more, you *are* going to lose weight. Some people will after one week, some after two. Some will lose two pounds one week, then none the next. Some will stop losing weight after a while, because their metabolism has slowed to match the number of calories they are eating, so they will have to adjust—to increase the amount of exercise or, in some cases, to cut more calories to continue to lose. But over the long arc of time everyone will lose weight. The only variables are how fast and how much.

Take ownership of your exercise program by knowing this information before you start. Then along the way use the tools we equip you with to measure your progress to see if it's working for you. Every six weeks you will want to use the information you gather via your assessments to modify your program. Six weeks is enough time for the milk teeth of improvement to emerge and not so long that you waste time if your plan needs tweaking. If you go longer and wait a year to test again, you may waste a year. If you go shorter and test every week, the span is too brief for any measurable advancements to emerge and you'll lose motivation.

Success-o-Meter

Besides testing every six weeks, have other means to assess your progress. This keeps you real about your improvements, bolsters your motivation, keeps you diligent, and determines whether your plan requires any adjustment. Say you want to reduce your weight by ten pounds to increase your chances of being able to complete a marathon. You will start with a realistic goal: Lose two pounds a month, starting six months in advance. (Not so realistic: Planning to lose that much weight starting *three weeks* before the marathon. If you cut back calories too dramatically while exercising, your body will consume the lean body mass you are working to build.)

As you train for the marathon, after a month to six weeks you will monitor your weight, note your progress compared to your six-week goal, and make adjustments if necessary. You will also keep track of your diet. If after two months you have not achieved your two-month weight-loss goal, you will determine why. Have you been consistent? Or have you been following the plan one day, then going to eat pizza and drink three beers the next? If consistency is the problem, then you know your solution: Redouble your efforts at consistency. On the other hand, if everything has been going in the right direction but a realistic weight loss has not been achieved, then you might want to try a stricter diet, for a few weeks at least, to jump-start your weight loss. (See "Max's Jump-Start Weight-Loss Diet" in Chapter 5.)

If your goal is to improve your performance, say, in swimming, cycling, running, or walking, you will want to break up that goal into what is realistic to achieve in six weeks. Then every six weeks, test yourself by measuring your time, power, or speed at three different perceived intensities: at a very weak pace, at a moderate pace, and at a very strong but not maximum pace. (More on this in Part Two.) If you have not achieved your goal, again, try to determine whether you have been consistent, or need to make other necessary adjustments.

Remain positive if these interim tests show that you have to modify your goals, and get excited about your new, more realistic ones.

Keep Your Program Individual

> Before Max gave us training programs as part of the 7-Eleven team, we all trained together. It was when we got *individual* programs that our talent began to develop.
>
> —Eric

Your parents were right: Just because your friends are doing something, it doesn't mean you should do it, too. Exercise is no longer a guessing game, no longer the province of conjecture and anecdote. ("Hey, it worked for him—maybe I should try it.") Physicians, scientists, and trainers have slowly and meticulously mapped the relatively new biological terrain of exercise physiology and continue to do so. Listen to them. Some medical studies on exercise have offered surprises.

One of the discoveries is that exercise programs need to be individualized. There is comfort in numbers, but you will experience improvement only by sticking with the program designed for you. Because the ideal exercise program is based on your individual starting point and your particular goals, it stands to reason that for you to be successful your exercise needs to remain focused and individual as well. Everyone wants to do what their friends are doing, however. So go out and have fun with them! But exercise with those who have very similar starting points and goals. When you take a yoga or karate or aerobic dance class or join a riding or running or walking club, the group is almost always divided up by ability; this is good. Likewise, you need to seek out people of the same ability to exercise with when outside organized groups. If you go on the group run or ride with your friends, you still must stick to your own prescription for the day (by going shorter, longer, or at an intensity different from that of the group if necessary). Or exercise with your friends exclusively on days when your programs happen to be in sync.

Don't Mix Programs

Along the way, resist the temptation to throw in training techniques from other programs. Every month all the fitness magazines run new programs for readers to sample. Limit your interest in these programs to your armchair. Don't graft on to your program a weight-training regimen from a running magazine or intervals someone at the gym does. We understand how these hodgepodge programs happen: A movie star says she's losing weight following the X program, and suddenly everyone's on the X program. Then next week, a high-profile athlete announces he's using the Y program, and so everyone adds ideas from the Y program.

Combining exercise programs is like merging diets, adhering to a low-carb diet for the main course and then a high-carb diet when dessert is served. People tend to cherry-pick the parts of programs that are most appealing at the moment, which may eliminate all of the complex cause-and-effect built into each plan. Switching programs midstream likewise may dilute or nullify the effects of either program.

The broader picture reveals that different people can achieve their best result with any one of a number of programs. There are many good options. However, there is no option when it comes to sticking with what you've started. To be successful, *you need to stick to one*, ideally the one that you can most closely tailor to yourself as an individual.

Meanwhile, do resist mixing or switching, even if you discover midway through Week 3 that some guy shooting hoops with you down at the park did it differently. His starting point could be completely different from yours, and his goals could differ wildly from your goals. Instead, stick to your program for at least twelve weeks. It takes six weeks for improvement to be readily measurable and for you to understand the minor adjustments you need to make, and three months for your body to develop and give you a true indication of whether the program is working. It's a big time commitment, which is why you want to pick a good program to start with.

The terrific thing about your goals is their plasticity: They will grow as you grow. You are, in a deep sense, a product of your goals. And how do you reach them? As you're about to see, through careful and methodical building.

"Our body is a machine for living. It is organized for that, it is its nature. Let life go on in it unhindered and let it defend itself, it will do more than if you paralyze it."

—LEO TOLSTOY

3

better foundation

Why does fitness improvement require so much planning, precision, and time? Because you are building a machine. First, you need to retool your systems for exercise; your body needs to construct the aerobic and strength-building machine. You now know that this work is a vast undertaking, reaching down to the intracellular level. Some systems take longer than others to be built, hence the reason you experience plateaus and the leaps in improvement. Once the systems have developed and the machine is complete, *then* each of your systems starts to sync up with the others and to chug along in unison. You will go from feeling as if you are pushing a 1950s Cadillac around the track to steering your new, souped-up ride effortlessly through the turns. Once you are running on all cylinders, you can move from building to *improving* the machine. That's when you will start to fine-tune, to add power and speed.

Sequencing

To achieve that level, however, the right exercise has to occur in the proper sequence. Some types of exercise or ways of doing exercise help build your systems. We give you these in the beginning or foundation-building phase of your program if you're just starting out. Other kinds of exercise help strengthen your systems; these we recommend in the strengthening phase. Still others are ideal for maintaining fitness. These you will do in the maintenance phase. In all phases, you want to follow each step; never skip ahead. Fitness is like building a house. First the soil must be tested, then the foundation poured. After that the frame is erected, and the roof, subfloor, Sheetrock, wiring, and plumbing are all added in the correct order. Retooling the human body for fitness is similar. If you work on the wiring before the walls are up, you can guarantee you will have problems.

Challenge Yourself Wisely

The sequence of exercise is a key concept. Your body also has to be challenged. We call this overload. Overload is not "no pain, no gain," and it's not going to the gym or the track and working out like crazy. Every time you place a greater-than-normal physiological or psychological demand on your body, you are generating overload. When those demands happen in an organized sequence—over and over again on a regular basis—that constitutes training. Overload is formally defined among training scientists in many ways, but we prefer to describe it as an organized and targeted structure of physical or psychological stressors designed to improve physical performance. That is, a fitness program.

Training overload makes you fitter by stimulating your body to adapt. These adaptations increase your body's ability to respond to stressors, physical or mental. For exercise to kick-start those improvements, it has to challenge you. We all know that to achieve anything in life (in school, at work, and so on) we have to work hard. Eric's credo is "If you want to be a champion you have to train like a champion." Seems simple enough. But somehow we equate exercise with play. Even people who exercise hard tend to favor certain activities—generally those that favor them. In other words, we tend to do what comes easiest to us. People with good cardiovascular fitness do aerobic activities. Those with muscular strength like to lift weights. Logically, we are attracted to the areas where we will receive the most immediate gratification. It's nice to do something you're good at. But now that you are enlisting your brain in the pursuit of fitness, you need to be aware of your tendency to do that, and try to choose activities that challenge you instead.

This is difficult when you are good at one kind of activity and bad at another. In truth, many people who have focused too long and hard on one area of fitness cannot tolerate other areas. Runners and cyclists often don't like to lift weights, even if they know that it could be beneficial. On the other hand, some weight lifters cannot tolerate walking a mile. It's actually painful for them. But having a diversified exercise portfolio, if you will, is necessary for a balanced fitness.

"Take" Exercise Regularly

"But I already have overload in my life," our patients say. "I play basketball every Tuesday night."

We all know a weekend warrior—someone who goes all out once a week or so but somehow never gets fit. There's a reason weekend warriors don't see huge gains in their fitness. There are two kinds of overload: chronic overload and acute overload. You go out today and run a half hour. That's acute overload. Your body will show response to that acute exercise: your heart rate goes up, your body temperature rises, you get some buildup of lactate in your muscle, you breathe faster. But when you stop, within minutes or hours the effect of that acute exercise is gone and your condition goes back to the starting point. Your body does not develop stable adaptations to acute overload or to stressors that occur only once, or only now and then. That's why you don't see much improvement from working out or doing an activity infrequently, why you don't get aerobically fit running after your kids for a few minutes, or get ripped with muscles after a day of moving.

Chronic overload, however, means *recurrent* stressors, performing the same challenges over and over again. You walk, you ride, you use the Stair-Master, or run for a half hour a day, three to five times a week for a month, or you lift weights three times a week. That's chronic overload. The human body has an incredible ability to adapt to chronic overload. Chronic exposure to overload is what makes you fitter, healthier, stronger; after a certain amount of chronic overload, you will start to see adaptations.

How Your Body Adapts

The adaptations your body produces in response to recurrent stresso can be either anatomical or functional. When you lift weights, you an anatomical change: You increase your muscle size. You also functional adaptation: You can perform the function of l weight, or the same weight more times.

Functional adaptations make the most of your po built with so much more potential than your daily stories in the newspaper about a mother who lifts the car off her child. Her body contains the muscle fiber to do that. Combined with the adrenaline rush, which focuses her mind to send a strong command to her muscles, she is able to lift the car, to compel her muscles to function together in one tremendous symphony of action. Without the command from her brain to recruit those muscles in the right way, however, it isn't possible to coerce them to function at their maximum potential. To utilize your maximum potential, your brain needs to better recruit the muscle fibers you need for any given action. Your brain needs to know not only which muscle fibers to contract but which opposing muscle fibers to *relax* to create a precise function. This is why weight lifters pause to focus before they lift, to consciously focus. You reinforce functional adaptations through repetitive experience. Read: practice.

Other modifications that result from recurrent stressors include increased blood flow to muscles due to capillary development as well as changes on the cellular level. (More on this in Chapter 4, "Better Strength.") When the recurrent stressor is an aerobic effort such as running or biking longer than a few minutes, you challenge your aerobic system—your heart, your lungs, and the energetic mechanism that utilizes oxygen. A brief effort like lifting a chair doesn't require much oxygen—we don't get out of breath. But during longer muscular efforts, your muscles require oxygen to produce energy. Thus, longer efforts develop your ability to dole out oxygen to every part of your body. If you do that often enough and long enough, you make better use of the air you breathe. To see these benefits, however, you need to commit a certain amount of time to aerobic activity at a certain rate.

Exercise at the Right Intensity

e more quickly triggered when you do exercise at the right

the temperature setting when you put food in the oven. mperature gauge when driving your car. When you head xercise, you also need to be aware of the temperature—the ich you exercise your body.

rives on precise doses; your body is, after all, a complex nd electrical impulses, which you can tweak to optimize as prescriptions and over-the-counter medications have you need to administer exercise at the right intensity to you desire.

You measure exercise intensity by your speed or your heart rate or the amount of weight you are lifting. That tells you how hard your system is working. (We will show you several ways to measure your intensity in Part Two.) Measuring intensity is easy, and you may do it already. But the importance of intensity is underestimated. It's easier to focus on time, miles, or repetitions. Thus, people have gotten into the habit of thinking about exercise in terms other than intensity. "I did thirty-five minutes on the treadmill today," they say. Even the surgeon general has contributed to this because he stated that people need "thirty minutes of moderate exercise most days of the week." What you hear is "thirty minutes." That is easy to define and understand. The intensity he recommends, moderate, on the other hand, is very general, and it means different things to different people.

When you talk about miles or time or repetitions, you are describing volume. Volume is important. It is one of the five parameters to consider when exercising—but only one of five. (The other four are intensity, frequency, density, and rest. You can turn the dial on any one of these to change your body's response to exercise.) Intensity is often *more* important than volume, especially when you cannot adjust volume due to the time limitations of family, work, civic obligations, and so on. Moreover, volume alone does not give a full picture of the level of biological stress you are putting on your body. For example, a runner will come into our office, and we'll ask him to give us a snapshot of his training.

"I'm running around thirty-five miles a week and I take one day off," he'll say. That means something, certainly, but in terms of evaluating the level of stress he is putting on his body, we don't know if he is doing thirty-five miles by going out on Sunday and pushing himself hard for twenty miles with a group, then running five miles every second day during the week at a very easy pace. Or if he does around six to seven miles every day at very high intensity, including track speed work.

For us, a picture of his week that included intensity would provide a more meaningful picture: "I run thirty-five miles and of those thirty-five miles, I have one long run when I run below my marathon pace or at my marathon intensity, and then a couple of days I do intervals at a submaximal pace."

You can appreciate that running five miles at high intensity is quite different from walking five miles. Keep in mind the importance of intensity with regard to your own exercise.

Learn to Listen to Your Body

Some programs do recognize the value of intensity, but they usually urge intensity based on a level or percentage of what you can do if you go all out, if you exercise at your maximum ability or intensity. If someone wants to improve her endurance, for example, a program will typically recommend that she exercise at 60 to 70 percent of her maximum heart rate. But there are some people who can sustain a higher percentage without causing an overload, and others who would suffer and be unable to sustain the activity at 50 percent of their maximum heart rate. Are their bodies experiencing the same workout at 60 to 70 percent of their maximum? Hardly.

We recommend instead that you target the intensity of your exercise based on how you perceive the exertion, and that you calibrate intensities starting from the bottom of the effort ladder (nothing at all; very, very weak; very weak; weak; moderate; and so on), and never actually reach your maximum. We have found it's not necessary.

You can take this a step further and mark down your heart rate as you work your way up the ladder. This is a way to target exactly what exercise is doing for your heart, your lungs, and your circulatory system. (We'll also show you how to do that.) You'll want to count the miles or the time or weight, too—perhaps those things make for better bragging—but what helps you biologically is tracking the *intensity*.

People see athletes wearing heart-rate monitors or counting their heartbeats while working out and assume that's something for elite athletes. The truth is, they are monitoring the intensity of their workout—making sure that they aren't doing "heavy duty" exercise when they need to do "medium" or "easy" exercise and vice versa. This is even *more* important to novices than to the elite. When you are starting out your body is still a bit delicate, so you want to monitor your body and be as precise as possible. And no matter your level, you get more out of your training when you are aware of the intensity of your exercise.

Exercise intensity is not discussed much because it's not simple. It's hard to sum up in a magazine article and impossible to apply to an entire Spinning or aerobics class. Any quick, blanket explanation cannot encapsulate it all. There's no magic intensity that works for everyone. You have to find the right intensity for you as an individual—and that, too, changes as you progress. But we'll show you how to do all of that.

"Take" the Right Amount of Exercise

We all know plants need water. But if you give a plant too much water, you're going to kill it. And some plants need more water; some need less.

Most people train hard when they take up exercise; they have a very strong work ethic and sense of commitment. They definitely cause overload. But they tend to focus more on going hard, and less on allowing for progressive increases. Instead, they exercise the first day and go until they drop. The next day they try to exercise even longer or harder. Then they are beat up for days.

This is not necessarily the best way to get from Point A to Point B.

Biologically, your body needs time to adapt to the training load. An athlete can actually shut down her body's adaptation process by exercising too hard, by not allowing a progressive increase in overload, and by not giving her body time to respond and adapt. The foundation of progressive overload is *gradual* change, to give your body time to respond to the stressors. You can't lift or run 5 percent more each day. Your body does need to be challenged by greater and greater amounts of exercise, but it also requires time off to adapt. If you train only once a week, that's not regular enough to expect any benefits. You may get the same effect if you increase too quickly or too often—that is, no effect. People often increase their training too quickly because they want to double up the payoff, but they actually delay the payoff, or quit or get injured. Or, if they stick with their program through the fatigue, they often end up with lower performance. Restrain those desires to do more right out of the gate, and you will do better in the long run.

Allow Rest and Recovery

A prescription antibiotic doesn't do its work while you're swallowing the pill—it does its work *after* you swallow it. Exercise is similar. The adaptations—the improvements—occur not while you're exercising but after the workout, when you are resting, during recovery. Once your body stops funneling resources to fuel exercise, it channels them for use in repairs. When it repairs, it adapts.

No matter how dedicated you are or how seriously you train, you need a certain period of time to allow your body to recuperate before stretching again to reach a higher level. It's impossible to go straight there.

—Greg LeMond
Three-time Tour de France winner

Rest and recovery are a fundamental part of an exercise program. The idea is to fatigue your body to a certain point, then give it a day or more of easy work so your body can experience what we call supercompensation—the anatomical and physiological changes that occur when you adapt to overload.

If you have failed at getting fit in the past, perhaps you've perceived a limit in your body, your mind, or your genes. Then again, what seems a limit may only be a limit within one small arena or activity; perhaps you haven't tried all the potential adjustments and options.

To be world class at any sport, you've got to be born with the right tools. Second, you've got to have the right frame of mind. There are a lot of people with the right tools, but they just don't have the drive. I had the drive to pursue speed skating and I found a sport that I was good at. If I'd gotten into cycling, I would just be another has-been.

—Eric

NOTE: In 1985, Eric became a national champion in cycling; a year later he competed in the Tour de France.

The evidence is overwhelming: The foundation of a successful exercise program is individualization because each athlete responds differently to various activities, training loads, and recovery time. When we train people and dial in the right sequence of chronic overload, intensities, and rest, they get worse for a while, yes, but then they get better. You, too, will tinker with choosing the right activities, keying into your perceived exertion, setting your exercise intensities, and noting your rates of adaptability. You will get fatigued and then you will get strong. You will get very strong. And you will be in control of the process, a process that takes place beneath your level of consciousness, in your circulatory system and muscles, which is the basis of your strength.

"Breath is life, and if you breathe well you will live long on Earth."

—SANSKRIT PROVERB

4

better strength

Everyone understands that muscles benefit from exercise. Their achievements are visible: flat abs, steely glutes and biceps. Less visible but more significant are the vast victories you experience elsewhere in your body. Exercise is a particularly potent prescription for your lungs, heart, and blood. You upgrade these when you do aerobic exercise—any activity that uses large muscles in a rhythmic way, such as running, walking, cycling, dance, swimming, and so on.

You breathe in, you breathe out, your heart beats, your blood flows. You don't really need to think about this much. So what's to improve? A lot. The truth is, with a little movement, your breathing, your lungs, your heart, and your blood become breathtakingly better. And with these improvements you can go from chugging along like a junker car to purring at top speed like a Ferrari.

These very real renovations start with your circulatory system. Every organ and cell in your body requires oxygen for life. The simplest single-cell organism takes oxygen directly from its environment. In more sophisticated animals—like us—the cells have specialized to perform different tasks, but each cell still needs oxygen. So we had to develop a system to bring oxygen from our environment to every cell; we do that via blood pumped by our heart.

Your heart delivers oxygenated blood to your cells via arteries, which divide off into passageways called capillaries that become smaller and smaller until they are the width of a single blood cell. After bringing oxygen and nutrients to each cell, these capillaries then connect with veins that race your blood back to your heart.

When you're active, you stress this system, and it beefs up in order to handle the new demands being placed on it. These improvements constitute a total remodel, upgrading every component of your oxygen-carrying system to state of the art, so that you can tote more oxygen to your muscles. Such comprehensive improvements are what convey the tremendous sense of well-being—that Ferrari feeling—that comes with fitness. Developing them requires time and exercise, however. To understand and appreciate what you have to look forward to, why you need aerobic exercise, and why you don't get fit over the weekend, you need to know how the components of your circulatory system improve.

Your Lungs

Better circulation starts with your lungs. Your lungs don't grow bigger or harder with exercise like your muscles do, but with exercise your lungs perform the same work using less energy. It's almost as if your lungs get smarter.

Exercise also spawns greater efficiency in moving air in and out of your chest, and in exchanging oxygen and carbon dioxide with your blood. Trained athletes tend to breathe slower and deeper. This reduces what's called the "functional dead space" in your lungs. This dead space resides in the tube between your lungs (where oxygen is transferred to your blood) and your mouth (where you get oxygen from the environment). If you have ever inhaled air through a snorkel, you know that it's harder to breathe. That's because the snorkel extends the dead space between your lungs and the air. You have to put more energy into sucking air in and out to move all of the air in the snorkel. Only the air that makes it deep into your lungs will bring oxygen to your blood, but you have to move all of the air in the tube to get new air down there. When you are active and need oxygen pronto, your body quickly realizes that dealing with the dead-space air between your lungs and mouth is like breathing through a snorkel. When you breathe faster, you have to suck in the air that's not contributing—that dead-space air—more times. You quickly discover that breathing slower and deeper is easier than breathing faster.

Dead-space air constitutes about a third of each breath you take in resting conditions. For every breath you can save, you reserve the energy it takes to move that amount. When resting, you suck in that useless air ten to sixteen times a minute. When you are aerobically fit, you draw it in fewer times a minute. That totals more than a quart of useless air you avoid sucking in *every minute*. Imagine a quart-size balloon filled with air and the energy it would take to suck that air out. That's the amount of energy you save every minute when you are fit, and you save even more while exercising.

This savings in respiratory work following training is substantial. Research demonstrates that when exercising at the upper limit you spend up to 8 percent of your total energy *just on breathing* (expanding your lungs and so on). The energy you save with better breathing is total gain; your body sends some of that energy to other muscles that are working hard, like your leg muscles. Thus by breathing deeply and less frequently, any given activity—walking, running, dancing, or swimming—is easier for you to do. You can sustain it longer; you feel less fatigue.

Another change in the breathing technique of fit people is that they keep less air in their lungs at the end of each breath. Basically they squeeze out more air. The changes in pressure that happen inside the chest during the respiratory movement help your blood return to your heart, favoring your circulation. With training, your respiratory pattern changes. Think of marathon runners: They are always relaxing their breathing. Their shoulders drop; each exhalation is very deliberate; they become veritable exhaling machines. This is an automatic, unconscious breathing pattern that allows for more air to come in at each new breath. This washes out more carbon dioxide (and you produce a lot of carbon dioxide when you exercise). It is, in a sense, a recyclable that gets tossed out at the energy factories in your muscles. At your muscles, blood delivers oxygen and picks up carbon dioxide, then returns to your lungs to dump carbon dioxide and retrieve fresh oxygen. When carbon dioxide accumulates, your blood becomes more acidic. It can't pick up as much carbon dioxide at the cells—and what it does pick up it can't drop off at the lungs. By exhaling more deeply when you exercise, you are washing out more carbon dioxide from your lungs with each breath.

Training benefits circulation even more. When you're fit, your lungs open up their "spare rooms," so to speak, so you use more of your lungs for air exchange. When you exercise you also distribute both the blood and the air in your lungs more evenly. At rest, when you are standing, a lot of blood stays in the basement of your lungs (due to gravity); most of the air keeps to itself at the top of your lungs, or in the attic, as it were. If you lie on your back, the same thing occurs—you have more blood at the back of your lungs, more air on top. When you exercise, however, the balance shifts and the two mingle better. They both filter into all of the rooms on all the floors of your lungs, in more equal proportions. This way, more blood comes in contact with more oxygen, and your blood is essentially better oxygenated when it returns to the heart and is pumped to the rest of your body.

Your Heart

Your heart becomes bigger *and* more efficient when you exercise regularly. Specifically, your heart's left ventricle—the part that pumps blood out to your body—holds more blood. The average adult left ventricle holds about 120 milliliters of blood, about half a cup. And that ventricle squeezes out between 55 and 60 percent of what it can hold—sixty-six to seventy-two milliliters of blood, a little over a quarter of a cup. Someone who exercises regularly, however, pumps out more—generally above 65 percent of what the left ventricle holds. That means that when you exercise, your heart squeezes out eighty milliliters of blood—a teaspoon to a tablespoon more than average—with every beat.

This adds up. A normal person in a resting condition pumps about five liters of blood to her body every minute, about a gallon and a third. When she's working out at maximum effort, she can expect to pump about three times that—between fifteen and eighteen liters per minute, or four gallons. An athlete in top condition pumps *twice* that—between thirty-five and forty liters per minute, or eight gallons per minute. That's an additional four gallons of blood pumped every minute. As a result, when you exercise you increase the amount of blood delivered to your muscles, and as you get fitter you deliver even more.

With exercise, the wall of your left ventricle thickens proportionally to the increase in the chamber's size, which renders a stronger ventricle. When your arm muscle gets stronger it can lift more weight; when your heart muscle gets stronger it can pump more blood with fewer beats. That's why trained athletes have a lower heart rate—their hearts are literally bigger and stronger. And like any other muscle, your heart muscle gets fatigued, but your bigger, stronger heart will pump more blood, and do so longer, with less fatigue.

Your heart's stroke volume is the amount of blood it pumps out with each beat. As with your breathing and lung volume, as you exercise you reduce the frequency of your heartbeats but increase the stroke volume. There are great advantages to this. The blood vessels that feed oxygen to your heart work mainly when your heart is relaxed, between pumps. Each time your heart beats, it squeezes shut those blood vessels, so the heart itself does not get blood or oxygen. When your heart relaxes, blood floods through those vessels and your heart feasts on oxygen once again.

The relaxation phase of a beating heart takes up two-thirds of each cycle, the contraction about one-third. This means your heart gets oxygen 70 percent of the time and is deprived of it 30 percent of the time. When you start to exercise, in the beginning your heart rate goes up and the contraction phase now takes up *half* your heart's time. Now your heart is getting oxygen only 50 percent of the time. That is quite a challenge for your body, especially when you consider that your heart's need for oxygen increases sharply with exercise. The increased demands placed on the untrained heart early in an exercise program coupled with the reduced amount of time the heart itself gets blood are among the reasons why exercise can produce symptoms for people with silent heart disease. As you continue to exercise, however, your body naturally regulates your heart. As your heart grows and thickens and pumps a greater volume of blood per beat, it accomplishes so much more with each beat that it no longer needs to beat as often. Your heart rate goes down. With fewer beats your heart has fewer contractions and that means less time your heart is largely deprived of blood and more time it enjoys full circulation. With a lower heart rate, your heart enjoys a lot more oxygen. For this reason, you need to start exercise slowly and build gradually to give your heart time to *build a better system*.

Your "Second Heart"

Didn't know you had a second heart? You do. Your heart pumps blood to the outer limits of your body, but your blood returns to your heart primarily through the squeezing action of your muscles, often referred to as your second heart. With exercise your muscles squeeze better and send more blood back through your veins to your heart. The amount of blood your muscles can return to your heart determines how well you refill your left ventricle, and that determines how much blood gets pumped to your body.

When your second heart is not functioning, your left ventricle doesn't refill adequately and thus your heart cannot supply adequate blood to your body. To imagine this at its extreme, think about a bridesmaid in a wedding party or a soldier in formation who faints. When forced to stand completely still for prolonged periods, your second heart isn't functioning. A quantity of blood remains in your lower extremities due to gravity. With less blood being returned to your heart, the ability of your heart to fill diminishes, and consequently so does its output. Less blood is pumped to your extremities, your organs, and your brain. And this situation can cause blood pressure—and the bridesmaid—to drop.

> When I was in the military as a young man and had to stand for long periods of time, I kept contracting my calves by performing little heel lifts. I did so and I never dropped.
>
> —Max

Capillaries

When you exercise, your capillary network, which carries oxygen to your muscles, also expands. A capillary is the smallest, most distant part of your arterial system. If your arteries were freeways, your capillaries would be the driveways to the cells, and in these driveways oxygen is delivered right to the doorstep of your cells and carbon dioxide is swept away.

An average person has one capillary for every five to fifteen muscle fibers. The people who do the most aerobic activity in the world—top endurance athletes—have one capillary for *every* muscle fiber. This brings each muscle fiber much closer to blood, so each one gets better oxygen delivery and better carbon dioxide disposal.

We all know that exercise lowers blood pressure, yet another benefit to your body's hydraulic system. Any fluid in a hydraulic system moves from a point of higher pressure to a point of lower pressure. To push your blood, your heart has to produce enough pressure to offset the lower pressure downstream in your capillaries. If pressure rises downstream in your capillaries, your upstream blood pressure has to climb as well, to allow the whole system to work. But if the pressure downstream eases, so can your upstream blood pressure. Since exercise adds virtually miles of capillaries, it's as if a million alternate routes become available on an overcrowded roadway. This gets your blood speeding along at the limit and lowers the pressure. The extension of new capillaries even offsets the increase in blood volume that is also created by exercise. (More on this later.)

The distribution of your blood is also upgraded. When you exercise, your body learns to do triage and send more blood where it's needed most at any given moment. This priority system works via a bypass or shifting mechanism. When you're fit and you, say, start running, this bypass shifts your blood away from muscles you aren't using and sends it primarily to the muscles you require to run. When you are unfit, your bypass system is not activated. Your brain gets the signal that the muscles in your legs need more oxygen, but your body has no ability to send blood primarily to your legs so your circulatory system floods your entire body with blood. Your face flushes, your head pounds, your heart races to keep up with this extreme demand, and your leg muscles—since they are not getting priority delivery—run out of oxygen very quickly. Exercise teaches your circulatory system to target the muscles that most require increased circulation, and not to randomly flood your entire body.

Better Blood

When you are challenged by any activity, you have yet another distinct advantage if you are fit: Your blood volume actually expands. You produce more red blood cells plus more plasma, the liquid that holds the cells in suspension.

You increase both red blood cells and plasma, but the amount of plasma increases by a greater proportion, which thins your blood. Thinner blood is easier to push through the capillaries, which as we said are very, very small (about one blood cell wide). Thinner blood means oxygen reaches farther out into your capillaries with less effort. Imagine drawing water up a straw. Easy, right? How about drinking a milk shake through the same straw? No doubt a milk shake requires more work than water. In the same manner, when you have the thinner blood of an athlete, you ease the work your heart has to do.

More blood makes life easier for your heart in another way, due to improved refilling. Think of two water balloons—one overfilled and one underfilled. Which one would produce a stronger stream of water if squeezed? When your heart fills to overfilling, it can push blood out with greater gusto.

Meanwhile, exercise is also a prescription for enriching that broth you send to your cells by increasing the number of red blood cells, but also by boosting each cell's share of hemoglobin. Hemoglobin is the compound that carries the oxygen in your red blood cells. The higher a person's level of hemoglobin, the better their potential aerobic performance. The effect is so dramatic that elite athletes sometimes turn to performance enhancement techniques that attempt to artificially bump up their hemoglobin mass through EPO (erythropoietin), blood transfusions, and other illegal performance enhancers. A legal option includes living in the mountains, at elevation, to naturally increase your hemoglobin mass, which is one of the steps that speed skaters on the U.S. team did prior to the Salt Lake City Olympics. You can get some of that same effect naturally when you exercise.

Better Arteries

So we know that drawing water up a straw is easier than doing so with a milk shake. Now imagine trying to draw a milk shake up a straw narrowed by a hardened coating of plaque. This happens naturally to your arteries as you age. With exercise, however, you eliminate plaques that have built up in your arteries. The difference between drawing water up a wide straw and trying to suck up a milk shake through a narrower straw demonstrates how completely exercise overhauls your body's circulatory system.

Your increased capillary network and corresponding lower blood pressure also impact your arteries. They get more elastic when they have lower pressure inside. Think of a garden hose. When the water is barely flowing through it, the hose is easy to bend. When you turn up the water to its highest pressure, the hose becomes rigid and unbendable. The same happens to your arteries. But with activity—and lower blood pressure—your arteries soften and become more flexible.

Cell Upgrades

I used to think about the cellular adaptations while training— how my mitochondria were adapting, what fuel stores I was using, how the actin and myosin were making my muscles contract. This made me feel empowered and part of the process.

—Eric

Your brain and all of your other organs benefit from these changes; each of your cells need oxygen, and every cell gets better service because it is receiving oxygen more efficiently. In addition, within each cell, the enzymes important in using long-lasting energy—specifically, processing oxygen to burn fat and sugars—get a boost. Your exertions can last longer because you are better able to use the fuel we all have in great abundance (namely, fat). The mitochondria, the little energy plants within our cells, also receive a bump-up in density and size, and they learn how to use high-intensity fuel (lactate) better. So if you exercise at high intensity—the level at which you normally build up lactic acid—you are able to clear it from your cells more quickly.

The Catch

You have just read how exercise is a potent prescription for your respiratory and circulatory systems. But there's a catch: All of this remodeling takes time. It doesn't happen if you merely go for a walk now and then. You need to stick with an exercise program for three to six months before you start to feel real changes and benefits. Of course, the changes start to develop right away, but realistically it's three to six months before these changes become significant. If you exercise two times a week for maybe only an hour each time, it's going to take forever. You wouldn't take an antibiotic now and then and expect it to be effective. Exercise, too, has to be taken in the right amount, at the right intensity, and the right frequency to be effective. The right amount is about three to five times a week, four to six hours a week. People who are already exercising six hours a week and want to improve significantly have to add another four to six hours. When you start at zero and have not exercised for a long time, your aerobic improvement will be enormous. With very little exercise, you get *a lot* of improvement. If you exercise faithfully and wait it out while this elaborate construction project is set in motion and then completed, your entire circulatory system will work better, and your whole body will win.

More Strength

Among the big winners of your beefed-up cardiovascular grid is your muscles, and this is a good thing. No matter how you measure fitness improvements, you are essentially gauging whether each muscle is contracting stronger and longer than last time. This ultimately comes down to how much energy you produce and on the quality of your muscle fibers.

Any physical movement you execute requires muscle contraction and the energy to make that happen. So training your muscles to contract is half the challenge, and the other half includes training the sources of energy that supply your muscle contraction. The energy you use to supply your muscles comes from four different sources, and they all get markedly better the more you use them. Once you understand how your muscles are fueled, you will be better able to gauge your progress and your fatigue. You will also be able to use exercise of different lengths and intensities to accomplish your dream, be it losing weight, gaining endurance, or increasing power or speed.

A Lightbulb Goes On

All cellular activity, including muscle contraction, is fueled by adenosine triphosphate, or ATP, a nucleotide that resides in each of your cells. ATP is essentially a lightbulb that can be turned on briefly using energy it has stored. After that, stored energy burns out and needs to be recharged. There are three ways to do this:

1. through what is basically a battery close by called creatine phosphate
2. through a virtual propane generator just outside the cell—the glucose stored in your muscles *or*
3. by plugging into a wall outlet to tap into juice from a remote power plant, otherwise known as your aerobic system, which burns fat and oxygen

When you sprint for a cab, when you run to a base in softball, when you play tag with your kids, or when you start to exercise at high intensity, you are using the lightbulb's small supply of stored energy. How long can this stored energy sustain a burst like that? About eight seconds. If you want to engage in an effort that lasts longer than eight seconds, your lightbulb will tap into the "battery" stored nearby. That battery is actually a compound called creatine phosphate; this will carry you for another two seconds or so.

If you run out of steam after ten seconds, does that mean you are a failure at exercise? Quite the contrary; these initial bursts can be lengthened somewhat with training, but they are limited to mere seconds for every human being on the planet.

Elite hundred-meter runners rely mainly on the lightbulb's stored energy and the nearby battery when racing, because they sprint one hundred meters in ten seconds. If you want to get fit for an activity like that, you might think you would never need to train the energy systems that kick in next. But most things in life take longer than ten seconds, including training for sprinting, so you need to push on.

If your cab takes off without you, you hit a triple, or your child is especially fast, you'll need another jolt of energy *immediately* to keep running. The glucose stored in your muscles—your "propane generator," if you will—now jumps in and powers the lightbulb for an additional forty seconds to two minutes. However, this produces a lot of lactate (essentially smoke), which is somehow linked to fatigue. When you see athletes who are performing at high intensity, you'll notice that they start to lose their form after forty seconds to two minutes; this means that lactate is building up in their muscles.

This generator propelling you now is burning glucose, converted from carbohydrates stored in your muscle. If you have been eating a low-carb diet, you will have little glucose stored in your muscle and your generator may sputter out early.

If one of your reasons for exercising is to burn fat, high-intensity exertions such as this won't torch that fat as well as other intensities. To burn the highest percentage of fat, you need to move to the next source: You need to plug your lightbulb into the wall, so to speak, and access aerobic energy, which essentially comes from stored fat and oxygen, the remote power plant with a virtually endless supply.

Energy that is aerobic (meaning "with oxygen") needs some ingredients that come from outside of your muscle; one ingredient is oxygen, supplied by your heart and lungs. This is used to burn fat and a varying percentage of glucose. Because aerobic exercise causes your muscles to move to burning *fat* in addition to glucose, it's the best type of exercise for weight loss. However, your exercise needs to last longer than a few minutes for fat burning to kick in.

If you decide to walk at this point instead of taking that cab, your aerobic system will definitely kick in. It will use oxygen to burn fat and glucose from your liver as well as what might remain in your muscle. Pure glucose, however, is your muscles' preferred fuel. As your body runs low on the glucose stored in your muscle, normally after forty-five to sixty minutes of exercise, and it switches over to a mixture that is a higher fat-to-glucose ratio, you'll experience a momentary sensation of being out of gas, of greater resistance, as if you're pushing through water. That's when athletes say they have "hit the wall."

Does *this* feeling signal you're completely out of gas? Not in the least. Your remote power plant can go virtually forever. It is essentially a low-volt source, so you won't be able to maintain the same high-intensity effort you could with the other sources, but it can propel you for a long time.

	POWER	CAPACITY
ATP	★ ★ ★ ★ ★	★
LACTIC	★ ★ ★	★ ★
AEROBIC	★	★ ★ ★ ★ ★

ATP: A lot of power for a very short period of time. Lactin (creatine phosphate): Allows you to maintain a pace four times as long. Aerobic: Supplies muscle and maintains pace for hours.

When you burn a mixture higher in fat, you are basically like a car running on a lower-efficiency fuel. For this reason, if you are planning to exercise for longer than an hour and a half, you need to restock your glucose stores along the way. Aerobic activity, especially endurance activity, does not work well for people eating a low-carb diet. At aerobic levels, they quickly run out of the glucose derived from carbohydrates, and feel empty and low energy.

Power Plug

Everything that affects energy delivery improves with training, including your brain and your liver. Even the way your DNA expresses different proteins depends on what you eat and how much you exercise. Exercise in general improves the amount of glucose you can store, in your muscles and in your liver, which improves your performance. Your brain (which uses a disproportionately high level of glucose) also benefits from this more constant supply of glucose. The more you exercise, the more you train the energy mechanism that powers you at your chosen level. For this reason, it's important to target your various sources of energy in an organized manner, to alternate stressing one energy system, then another, and allowing each one some relative rest. When you're starting out, aerobic activity trains all of the energy sources. But as you advance you will work on each system deliberately.

The most extensive change in your ability to produce energy occurs when you do aerobic exercise. As we said earlier, with aerobic exercise your mitochondria increase in size and number. In addition, the enzymes within your mitochondria get more efficient at producing energy. Your mitochondria also learn how to use lactate better. So even when you exercise at high intensity (when lactate normally builds up), you are able to clear it more quickly.

We find that aerobic athletes (cyclists and marathoners in particular) have far more mitochondria than average folks due to their training, up to 200 percent more. Mitochondria are important because the more you have, the higher percentage of fat you utilize at any given speed. Need more incentive?

When you're in poor aerobic shape, you have fewer mitochondria, and you don't churn through as much of your fat reserve as you could. Instead, you're running primarily on glucose, which means you'll run out of fuel faster. As you get into shape you increase the number and quality of your mitochondria. This ups the amount of fat you burn, which reserves your stored glucose longer, and you can also produce more energy for a longer period of time. (Even the most fit people in the world carry almost forty thousand calories in fat.) A side benefit of losing fat is that you dissipate heat easier, keeping your body cooler, which means you don't require as much water to keep your core temperature steady.

Jeff Pierce, the first American to win the Champs-Élysées stage of the Tour de France, knows the consequences of running low on carbs. In the Pyrenees, he missed grabbing his food bag, and it was clear to those of us in the support car that he was bonking bad: He was lethargic and had no energy. We got to be good at recognizing that—a rider sitting back, less reactive, dropping his cadence. We would ask, "Are you eating? Are you drinking?" The only thing I had in the car was a Coke. I handed it to Jeff out the car window. He started to drink it, the sugar started to take effect, and the next thing I know he was passing our car.

—Max

BURNING FAT

You burn the highest percentage of fat when you do moderate-intensity aerobic exercise. At rest, you burn approximately 50 percent sugar and 50 percent fat. When you run a 10k, you burn primarily glucose or sugar (about 99 percent). When you walk, you burn a higher ratio of fat (60 percent fat to 40 percent sugar).

THE ONE-MINUTE EFFORT	
ATP	40%
LACTIC	50%
AEROBIC	10%

In a one-minute effort, 40 percent of the energy comes from ATP, 50 percent from the lactic mechanism, and 10 percent from aerobic. In a marathon, 95 percent comes from the aerobic mechanism and 5 percent from the combination of ATP and lactic.

You burn the most calories when you go fast, but most of those calories are from sugar, and you cannot sustain the effort very long. When you exercise at moderate intensity, you burn the highest percentage of fat and you can go for a long time; however, moderate-intensity exercise doesn't burn as many total calories unless you go for a long time. If you want to burn fat, the trick is to find the balance of the greatest percentage of fat burning with the highest number of total calories burned for the amount of time you exercise. Here are a few general guidelines to maximize weight loss.

To lose weight (fat):

- If you can exercise for at least an hour, to lose the most fat you should exercise at moderate intensity. This will burn 60 percent of the total calories from fat, and the total calories burned will be significant enough to make a difference.

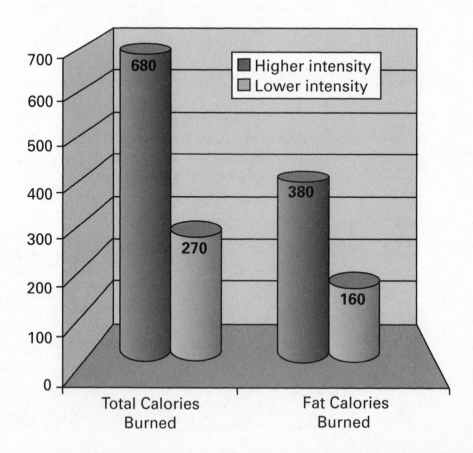

■ If you have only twenty minutes to exercise, to lose weight you need to go a little faster. At a higher intensity you will burn only 20 percent of the total calories from fat, but that 20 percent will equal more fat calories than if you went slow, got a 60 percent benefit, but burned fewer total calories.

For each individual there is an intensity and a duration at which he will burn the highest number of calories from fat. To determine this intensity precisely, you need to get tested at a lab. (For more information, see Part Two.)

Fast-Twitch vs. Slow

As we said earlier, when you exercise, your capillary network becomes more extensive, sending tributaries of blood closer to each muscle fiber. And the muscle cells themselves change by producing more of the enzymes important in processing oxygen to burn fat and sugar.

You train your muscles when you do any exercise, but they don't just get stronger, they get smarter, too. The muscles of your legs, arms, back, abdomen, and so on are made up of fibers—actually three kinds of fiber. One is small, or skinny, slow-twitch fiber. These are slow-contracting muscle fibers that use mainly oxygen. The second is fat, fast-twitch fiber. These fast-contracting muscle fibers don't use oxygen very well. The third is changeable: It can do the work of fast-twitch or slow-twitch fibers, depending on what is necessary, moment by moment or over a lifetime. Your muscles contain all three types.

Muscle fibers perform varied jobs. Not only do they have different physical characteristics, but they function differently, too. Picture an endurance athlete like a marathon runner. He doesn't bulge with muscle; he is hard and slender. That kind of activity favors people with a preponderance of skinny, slow-twitch fibers. On the other hand, picture a weight lifter or a sprinter; her activity requires fatter, fast-twitch muscle fibers. The leg muscles of the average adult are composed of about 60 percent slow-twitch fiber and 40 percent fast-twitch; the exact ratio is primarily determined by that of your parents. But some people have a higher ratio of one to the other. The leg muscles of a sprinter are 80 percent fast-twitch and 20 percent slow. A marathoner has 90 percent slow-twitch and 10 percent fast.

Our ratio of muscle fibers is also influenced by the kinds of exercise we do. That's why you don't see marathoners who look like weight lifters or sprinters, and you don't often see sprinters running marathons.

Fifteen to 20 percent of your muscle fiber is available to transfer from one type to the other, depending on the kind of training you do. For this reason, at the elite level, if an athlete does a lot of aerobic sports, it's a trade-off for some strength, and if they do strengthening exercise, they will lose some of their endurance. However, as mentioned, your ratio of dedicated fast-twitch fibers to slow-twitch fibers is largely genetically determined. If you have 90 percent slow-twitch fibers like a world-class distance runner, even if you train for ten years you'll never beat sprinters like Carl Lewis or Maurice Green, because you cannot change your genes, and you cannot change your physiology and your muscle fiber ratio that dramatically. This is true for everyone. In addition, as you get older, your fast-twitch fibers naturally become more slow-twitch. That's why you see people in their forties running their personal best in marathons, but never in sprints.

It is difficult for many people to understand why someone like Carl Lewis—a great hundred-meter runner—would never win a marathon. But now you can understand it just by looking at him: He has big, bulging muscles, while a marathon runner has long, skinny muscles. It isn't fair, but this is why it's important to choose ambitions that match your strengths, that are in keeping with your natural muscle composition. It is also important to exercise your areas of weakness, because this recruits those changeable fibers where you need them.

In any activity in life, you recruit muscle fiber going from smaller to bigger, depending on the amount of power required for your task. When you do an activity like cruising on a bike at low speed, you use small, slow-twitch fibers. You don't really need to apply a lot of force to the pedals, so you don't really need to wake up the big fibers. These slow-twitch fibers don't fatigue. You can go forever as long as you eat and drink.

When you start to go a little faster, which requires more force on the pedals, you recruit bigger fibers, and they fatigue at a faster pace. You may be able to sustain your tempo for thirty minutes to an hour, but then you'll be exhausted.

If you go all out—say you want to do your best mile—you recruit all three fibers, because you need all of them. But because the big fibers fatigue so quickly and create so much lactic acid, you are going to find yourself in a couple of minutes unable to keep working. Your muscles will be burning and you will be gasping for air.

Again, your muscle composition is primarily determined by that of your parents. If you want to know your ratio, you have three options: You can get a muscle biopsy for a precise measurement. You can guess—were you better at jumping high and sprinting, or at running for a long time? Or you can take the following test.

The Twitch Test

You can measure your ratio of fast-twitch to slow-twitch fibers by doing a vertical jump test, which measures the relative ratio of fast-twitch fibers your leg muscles contain. Those with a majority of fast-twitch fibers can jump higher. In the lab we use a force plate for this, but you can do it at home as well.

Mark a place on a wall as high as you can touch on tiptoes, using wet or chalked fingers. Next, again using wet or chalked fingers, jump as high as you can and touch the wall. Measure your best distance. If you are fit and can jump twenty inches or more above the highest spot you could touch standing still, you have a higher ratio of fast-twitch fibers. If you are fit and can jump eight to twelve inches, you do not have a high ratio of fast-twitch fibers. Of course, there is no way to say precisely the ratio without a muscle biopsy.

I was always better at sprinting than endurance. It's easier for me to do a sport that is about speed. I have a very high vertical jump, could play soccer, was good at sprinting. When running, I could outsprint all my friends, but I'm never going to win an endurance event. On the other hand, my wife, Julie, is a marathoner. She can go forever. She ran a marathon just nine months after our daughter, Sara, was born.

If we ever are chased by a bear, I have to hope he catches us quickly, because if the chase goes on for a while, I'm in trouble.

—Max

All of these improvements constitute the way in which exercise revolutionizes the Olympics of your daily life: lifting groceries, doing hobbies or home improvement projects, caring for children, concentrating at work, even sex. The more you demand of your body, the more your body will rise to the challenge and grant you the ability to do it.

That improvement revolution requires that you provide two elements: the right food and fluid to fuel it.

"A bear, however hard he tries, grows tubby without exercise."

—A. A. MILNE
AUTHOR OF WINNIE-THE-POOH

5

better fuel and fluids

Many people seek fitness to lose weight. Ten pounds, twenty-five pounds, a hundred pounds. It's important that you feel successful when getting in shape, and many people measure fitness success by weight. In addition, the fuel you give your body (in the form of food) has a significant impact on how successful you are at fitness. Food plays a powerful role in how well people feel and do athletically. Research, however, shows that among overweight people, many aren't getting what they need nutritionally. Many overweight people, ironically, are in want of vital nutrients. With low stores of vital nutrients, people don't have the energy to start exercising or the resources to build lean body mass. Even people who are very fit are uncertain about what to eat or drink and when. For these reasons, exercise cannot be addressed adequately without a serious look at nutrition.

In this chapter, with the help of our former colleague Marlia Braun, Ph.D., R.D., we will detail the facts that are known regarding the ideal ways to eat to fuel your body for fitness while also losing weight. Marlia has not only worked as the sports and health nutritionist for UC Davis Sports Medicine for eight years advising athletes of all ages, levels, and sports, she also draws upon her own experience as a world-class athlete.

Food as Fuel

A Formula One race car cannot be separated from Formula One fuel. Likewise, the food you eat cannot be separated from your body and its performance. Traditionally, in the medical community in the United States, nutrition has taken a backseat with regard to fitness. So important is the role of food in fitness, however, that in Europe all doctors trained in the specialty of sports medicine as Max was are also trained as sport nutritionists.

Over the last twenty years, as we've worked as physicians with athletes, we have also observed how powerfully food and hydration impacts how well people feel and do athletically. In fact, we think of nutrition—what food you eat and when you eat it—as a performance enhancer more effective and potent than any drug a pharmacist could prescribe. We are going to help you see why.

There are several behaviors you can easily adopt to ensure that your daily food intake will get you and keep you on track to a healthier, fitter body. These habits are easy and enjoyable. In many cases, the right nutrition for a fitter body is easier and more satisfying than bad eating habits.

In a nutshell, for optimal weight loss while embarking on a fitness program:

1. Eat every three to four hours.
2. Include protein in every meal to ensure that you're getting adequate amino acids and to keep you satisfied and alert until the next meal.
3. Add color (fruits and vegetables) at all meals and mid-morning and afternoon snacks.
4. Drink enough water so that you are urinating every two to four hours and your urine is relatively colorless and odorless.
5. To fuel your body for exercise and build lean body mass, eat a diet high in carbohydrates from fruits, vegetables, and dairy products.
6. Learn how to shop to keep healthy food handy.
7. Learn how to eat well at restaurants and parties.
8. Eat food to fuel your body, not to fulfill cravings.

Recipe for Weight Gain

Many people approach weight control by skipping food or eliminating food groups. They wait too long to eat, then overindulge later. They completely ignore their body's need for good fuel, then eat without regard for what their body needs, without consciously choosing the proper quantity, method of preparation, nutritional value, often without even being aware of when and why they are eating. By the time they turn their attention to fueling their bodies, they are so hungry they only care about satisfying the hunger, not supplying their body with the proper fuel. It's difficult to make good nutritional choices, do food prep, or eat moderately with this strategy. It's important that you don't avoid certain food groups, severely restrict your calories, skip meals, or ignore your hunger. We advise eating smaller amounts of *better* food with greater frequency instead.

Elite athletes approach food as fuel, pure and simple. Yes, it should taste good (otherwise you won't eat it and your body needs the fuel), but don't sacrifice nutritional value on the altar of tastiness. When you exercise, your body requires specific nutrients as building blocks to supply your rapidly adapting systems. Food packed with carbohydrates, protein, healthy fats, vitamins, and minerals provides the necessary parts to build and reinforce your developing muscles, and respiratory, cardiac, and nervous systems. Junk food—food that contains no or few valuable nutrients—delivers shoddy materials to your burgeoning systems, which means that sometimes your body is forced to scavenge nutrients from other areas of your body. The right food supports the time and effort you dedicate to exercise and to your goals. With healthier food choices, you'll reach those goals faster.

Food as a Prescription

Exercise is like a prescription medication; it has to be taken in the right amount at the right intensity on a regular basis to be effective. You need to eat prescriptively as well: the foods that serve the needs of your muscles, brain, organs, and metabolism. You can't let busy schedules and poor choices made in the heat of hunger override what your body really needs. When hunger calls, think prescriptively.

Eat Carbohydrates

Carbohydrates are essential for improving your fitness level; they supply energy to your muscles and your brain. Carbs have been demonized by diets that made the erroneous link between carbs and being overweight. The truth is that oversized portions and empty junk food carbs are the villains.

Carbs are not limited to potatoes and rice. Grains, fruit, vegetables, beans, and dairy are also carbohydrates. These foods also contain an un-digestible form of carbohydrate called fiber. You need fiber (25 to 30 grams a day) not only to prevent cardiovascular and colon diseases but to help you feel fuller between meals and snacks.

Carbohydrates also fill your glycogen pantry, the storeroom from which your body derives energy when you are exercising. And that means you will have the energy to exercise and that you won't succumb to those afternoon or evening snack attacks. You store carbohydrates in your liver and your muscles in the form of glycogen. You need to fill your glycogen, or carb pantry, even more when you exercise. People on low-carb diets often complain that they can't sustain their intensity or endurance like they once did. Indeed, when your glycogen stores are low, you hit the wall.

Eat Protein

Your muscles are made up of protein, so as you build lean body mass through activity you need protein. Protein is also necessary for your immune system, to produce hormones, and to repair and maintain all types of body tissues.

You actually have not one but many proteins in your body, and they each perform a different job. When you eat a food made up of protein, you break it down into its basic unit: amino acids. Then you build the specific proteins *you* need from those amino acids.

There are twenty amino acids you need in order to construct the various proteins your body requires to function. Eleven of these amino acids your body can build; nine, however, it cannot, so you need to eat them, in the form of animal products (beef, chicken, turkey, fish, eggs, and pork) and soy (tofu, soy milk, miso).

Some vegetarian sources of protein, such as beans (lentils, black, kidney, garbanzo) and grains (rice, pasta, polenta, couscous) are missing one or more of those nine amino acids. In fact, beans are missing one amino acid and grains are missing another. If you combine these two protein sources, however, you get all of the essential amino acids you need.

Protein (along with fiber) helps you feel awake and bridges the gap between meals. More, however, is not better. Protein supplements do not build more muscle, as some bodybuilding powders may claim. Eating more protein than your body requires each day, quite to the contrary, can affect your kidneys and liver, which process and excrete the nitrogen by-product of protein, and store what's left as fat. Choose lean protein and try to eat protein at each meal.

Eat Fats

Fat provides fuel during endurance activities (when your muscles burn fat) and aids in your body's use of vital fat-soluble vitamins. Certain fats also help you build a strong immune system, nerve fibers, and healthy skin; and reduce the inflammation associated with cardiovascular disease and cancer. These healthier fats include polyunsaturated fats and omega-3 and omega-6 fats from:

- Nuts
- Vegetable oils
- Flaxseed
- Fish

Another good fat, monounsaturated fat, can help you reduce your cholesterol and your risk of heart disease. Its sources include:

- Olive oil
- Avocado
- Peanuts

Fats to **avoid** include saturated fat (found in animal products), palm oil, coconut oil, and trans fat found in processed foods and snacks (identified on ingredient labels as partially hydrogenated oils). However, don't avoid all fats. Fats are just as important as vitamins and minerals. You will improve your fitness by consuming good fats in the right amount, about 30 percent of your total calories (that's about 3 grams of fat or 27 calories from fat for every 100-calorie serving).

Eat Vitamins and Minerals

Vitamins facilitate hundreds of biochemical reactions in your body that facilitate bone growth, healthy skin, and reduced oxidative stress. They also support carbohydrate, fat, and protein metabolism. Minerals serve in biochemical functions having to do with your bones and teeth, immune system, and oxygen transportation; and play critical roles in energy production and in your body's pH (acid) level and fluid balance. Minerals are abundant in food sources such as fruits, vegetables, and whole grains as well as dairy and lean meats.

Many people don't get adequate vitamins and minerals because their diet is made up of too many empty calories—foods that don't contain vitamins. It's difficult for your body to function, much less exercise, with inadequate vitamins and minerals. Potato chips and cookies don't contain vitamins and minerals; fruits, vegetables, and whole grains do.

To get adequate vitamins and minerals, eat from a wide variety of fresh foods. No multivitamin can take the place of real, whole food. Why do nutritionists always say this? There are nutrients, such as phytochemicals found in fruits and vegetables, which are not yet in pill form. If you eat a wide variety of fresh fruits and vegetables instead of relying on a pill, you are assured of not missing out on these important compounds. Vitamin pills also don't contain the fiber of whole foods. Aim to consume your vitamins and minerals by making each calorie in your diet count. (More on vitamins and minerals later in this chapter under "Supplements.")

Consume Fluids

Water is the most important nutrient. It's key to cellular function, transporting oxygen and nutrients, lubricating joints, eliminating waste, and maintaining your body temperature.

Your level of hydration can have a big impact on your success in initiating and maintaining a fitness program. When you are dehydrated you can feel dizzy, tired, thirsty, impatient, weak, and suffer headaches, all of which can bring your workday to its knees. If you get dehydrated while exercising, you may also suffer premature glycogen depletion; increased heart rate, body temperature, perceived effort, and stomach upset; decreased blood volume; and stomach emptying. Dehydration can also compromise your mental capacity and fine motor skills.

Your body is 50–65 percent water. A person who weighs 150 pounds is carrying around roughly 170 cups of water. You naturally lose about eight to ten cups (eight ounces each) of water a day, depending on how much you sweat and urinate. That's about 15 percent of your total water. Your brain is 75 percent water. Dehydration of your brain can result in a dull headache. When you suffer from a dull headache (after a busy day, or a long day outdoors exposed to high temperatures, which cause a loss of body fluids through sweat), examine your water consumption that day; you may need to drink.

Blood is nearly 60 percent water. If you lose more water than you consume, your blood can thicken, slowing its movement through your blood vessels. Your heart has to beat faster to move that thick blood so it can transport valuable nutrients and oxygen to your demanding cells. Have you ever gone out for an easy walk and felt winded, with your heart racing? You were probably dehydrated.

When you exercise, on average you sweat a little less than a liter to a liter and a half (three to six cups) per hour, but your stomach can absorb only eight hundred to one thousand milliliters of water (about three and a half to four cups) an hour. In other words, you cannot absorb as much as you can sweat. The key to making up for the deficit is to practice preventative hydration throughout the day so that your body has adequate water to support exercise later. Remember, fruits and vegetables are 95 percent water. So drink fluids with and between meals, and eat lots of fruits and vegetables.

How Much to Eat

You need a certain number of calories per day simply to live—to supply the basic functions of your heart, lungs, digestive system, brain, and muscles. Most adults need between 800 and 1,200 calories a day just to survive. Add to that additional calories required to fuel the level of activity you maintain each day. This is called caloric expenditure. Most people between thirty and seventy years of age need an additional 300 to 1,200 calories a day on top of their baseline 800 to 1,200. That's a total of 1,200 to 3,000+ calories a day, depending upon your job, body size, activity level, and other factors.

You consume calories (in the form of protein, carbohydrates, or fats) and they are either utilized or stored. When you consume more calories than you use, you gain weight. When you consume fewer calories than you use, you lose weight. The more you move, the more calories you require. To get a sense of how many more calories an hour of exercise burns, here are some examples: If you walk or bicycle an hour a day, you burn roughly 150 and 550 additional calories, depending on how much you weigh and how fast you go. If you jump rope for an hour, 500 to 1,000 additional calories are used up. If you jog, 600 to 1,200 calories.

Losing Weight

Again, to lose weight, you need to consume fewer calories than you burn. Seems simple, but it gets more complicated. At one extreme of the spectrum, seriously obese patients are put on very, very restricted diets of around 800 calories a day. That's about the equivalent of eating five apples a day. (We do not recommend eating five apples a day, by the way.) These patients lose weight very quickly in a short amount of time, but they suffer from dizziness, and other symptoms, because 800 calories is barely enough to supply their basic metabolic functions.

At the other end of the spectrum, an elite athlete who is training hard consumes between 4,000 and 5,000 calories a day; while competing in the Tour de France, a rider might eat as many as 8,000 calories a day just to maintain his body weight while sustaining extreme activity six hours a day. (They aren't just cruising, taking in the scenery, and they don't stop for food or water.) In fact, one of the major challenges of long-distance athletes is to maintain their caloric intake; as part of their training, they actually learn how to eat as a contestant. Most of us land somewhere in between the five-apple diet and the Tour de France requirements. In order to take control of your weight, you'll want to know how many calories you require, which will change as you become more active.

Pyramid Power

The U.S. Food Guide Pyramid Web site allows you to find out the number of calories and servings of each food group you should be eating for your age, gender, height, weight, and physical activity (www.mypyramid.gov). A lot of medical knowledge and expertise was brought to bear in creating the food pyramid and it's instructive to get a version tailored exactly to your needs and then compare it to the food and drinks you consume on a daily basis.

When I was training for the Olympics as a speed skater and as a cyclist for the U.S. championship, Tour de France, and other races, my diet was highly specialized, designed by a panel of experts. Ditto for when I was growing up. My panel of experts? The experts who put together the U.S. government's recommended dietary guidelines—the food pyramid. It's great free advice, but it's so simple and obvious many people don't appreciate how valuable it is.

—Eric

Document Your Diet

Once you know the number of calories you need to consume per day, you need to start comparing that benchmark to what foods in what quantities you eat per day. One way to do this is by keeping a food journal. Many people keep one for a couple of weeks and are shocked to discover how much they eat, how much they eat out, and how little they eat of certain food groups, especially fruits and vegetables. An honest food diary can offer insights that come as a big shock, especially to people who thought they were eating well, but it's hard to ignore the facts when they are tracked on paper. It's a very concrete way to chart what you've eaten and see the nutrients you're missing. It's also a great way to discern trends or unconscious eating patterns. If you want even more insight into your eating patterns, your food journal can also include daily exercise and other activities, energy and hunger levels, and calorie distribution.

Studies show that people who document their diet, on average, choose better food. They also have more success at losing weight and maintaining it long-term. There is definitely a sense of accountability when you have to document every morsel you munch. You will give certain foods a second thought when you have to admit to eating them on paper.

Take Food in Five Doses a Day

Quantity and type of food aren't the only factors that impact how your body stores or uses food; the timing of your meals is also relevant. We evolved from hunter-gatherers—from people who ate food as they found it, who didn't have to wait for their lunch break only to gobble down a candy bar and a bag of chips from the vending machine. Humans have not evolved to catch up with these busy lives or the conveniences of grocery stores and fast foods. Modern civilization, your work schedule, and your other obligations artificially dictate that you divide your food intake into three meals a day, but biologically, your body does better when you eat more often—about every three to four hours.

When you eat three meals a day, spacing your food consumption much more than three hours apart, your body perceives this period without food as a fast. The hunter-gatherer in you perceives this fast as "starvation!" and goes into emergency mode. This is especially problematic once you begin an exercise program. Your body also sees this emergency mode as a time to conserve energy. Your metabolism inches to a virtual halt and you start hoarding fat. When you finally do eat, the calories you consume are sent straight to the fat vault because your body thinks you're experiencing a famine and it needs to store as much as possible. Typically, if you wait this long to eat you will also overeat. Studies show that if you wait longer than five or six hours to eat, you consume disproportionately larger meals. Current research also reveals that smaller meals are the ticket to weight loss and maintenance.

Think Small and Nutritious

So the key to eating every three hours without overeating is to eat *small* amounts of *nutritious*, low-fat foods. Think small and plan ahead. Tactics include:

- Plan meals and snacks a few days ahead of time
- Cut in half the portion you would typically eat
- Savor the meal and make it last
- Leave the meal and snack not hungry but not full
- Make sure each meal features three food groups and the snacks have two food groups (this helps you feel more satisfied)

Go Back to Eating Fruits and Vegetables

Fruits and vegetables are good choices for every meal and snack. They're low in calories and high in nutrients. Many people stopped eating fruits and vegetables, along with pastas and rice, when the low-carb diet craze was in full swing and since then seemed to have forgotten these nutrient-rich necessities.

The U.S. Dietary Guidelines suggest seven to nine servings of fruits and vegetables a day—two to four servings of fruit, five of veggies. We hear from so many people, "How can I possibly eat that many fruits and vegetables a day?" The answer: By eating fruits or vegetables at every meal, including at mid-morning and mid-afternoon snacks. You need to drink them as juice and pack them to work as snacks. (Juices should be labeled 100 percent fruit juice, not "fruit drinks" or "fruitade"; and remember juices have less fiber than whole fruit.) Keep dried fruit handy for snacks on the move. When at a party or a buffet, choose celery sticks and broccoli flowerets over the baked Brie or chips. Chop fruit or veggies to pack as salad for lunch and slice fruit for dessert. Don't waste any eating opportunities by munching away on empty calories.

And watch your servings. A serving of fruit or vegetable juice is three-quarters of a cup, or six ounces (that's four shot glasses of juice—not a tumbler full). A serving of fresh fruit is eight ounces or half a cup. Our friend nutritionist Marlia Braun points out that industrialized farming techniques and hybrid varieties produce bigger fruit now. Apples used to be the size of tennis balls—one serving. Today, an apple can be three servings; a regular banana as large as one and half servings.

Fill Up on Fiber

The average American eats only 12 grams of fiber per day. However, women need to eat 25 grams per day and men 37 grams per day. Fiber helps control weight in several significant ways. First, high-fiber foods typically have a low glycemic index. According to the Harvard School of Public Health, diets that include many high glycemic–index foods, which cause quick and strong increases in blood sugar levels, have been linked to weight gain, as well as an increased risk for both diabetes and heart disease.

Fiber also gives you a sense of satiation by slowing down digestion and the uptake of carbohydrates into your blood. And by keeping yourself full you can more easily bridge the gap from one meal to the next. Fiber also has dramatic effects on your risk for cardiovascular disease by reducing your total blood cholesterol. Fiber can also reduce your risk for developing colon diseases such as constipation, diverticulitis, and colon cancer.

Increase your fiber intake by eating more raw fruits and vegetables (unpeeled when possible), and by eating more whole grains, such as whole wheat pasta and brown rice, as well as a variety of different kinds of beans.

Daily Fuel Prescription

There are specific techniques to consuming meals and snacks that we have found work well with athletes, including how to integrate the ideal protein, fiber, fluids, and healthy fats into your diet to assure adequate nutrient intake for strong physical performance.

Many sports nutritionists vote for a breakfast that contains 25 percent of your daily caloric needs. If your daily caloric needs are 1,200, your breakfast should be 300 calories; if your caloric needs are 2,400, then you need to consume 600 calories for breakfast, and so on. For most people 25 percent of daily intake is 400 to 500 calories. (Other nutritionists recommend eating a greater percentage of your calories earlier in the day, then reducing the size of each successive meal, until the evening meal, which should be light to avoid fueling your sleep.)

Breakfast is important because you need to fuel yourself for the day. You raid your inner pantry during the night, so it's particularly important to refuel your glycogen stores. In addition, if we're working with someone who has a job that does not allow for a break to eat a significant lunch, we recommend she eat a more substantial breakfast. If we're working with someone who doesn't work, we give him a light breakfast before he does his morning training and then a bigger breakfast after his workout. Altogether, his total caloric intake for breakfast, however, would still be 25 percent; it would just be split over two meals.

To start your day right, poised for exercise and activity, you definitely need to consume carbohydrates complemented with protein to slow digestion and the absorption of the carbohydrate. Also, drink two eight-ounce glasses of water. Wholesome and healthy breakfast choices for people who are exercising include:

- Multigrain cereal with milk or yogurt plus fruit
- Two scrambled eggs or egg substitute
- Oatmeal with berries and/or yogurt
- A smoothie with fruit, fruit juice, yogurt, and a scoop of protein powder
- A slice of whole wheat toast with peanut butter and jelly
- Whole wheat bagel with two eggs and one ounce of cheese

Morning Snack

Two to three hours after breakfast we recommend a snack along with more water. An ideal snack contains color and at least two different food groups. The focus is on carbohydrates to help keep your glycogen stores full, and fiber and protein to keep you satisfied until lunch. Good snack possibilities include:

- A cup of yogurt and a piece of fruit
- Four whole wheat crackers and an ounce of cheese
- A piece of fruit with a tablespoon of nut butter
- Dried fruit and nuts in a preportioned bag
- An energy bar (but not a meal replacement bar; they contain too many calories for a snack)

If you do not have a refrigerator close by or if you're in your car all day, equip yourself with a small insulated bag and a few freezer packs to keep fresh, healthy food handy.

Mix up the foods you eat; don't choose the same things day after day. Monday's snack could be a fruit salad. Tuesday's could be yogurt and an apple. Wednesday's snack could be a smoothie; Thursday's a strawberry with half a protein bar. Friday, eat cucumber like an apple.

Also, monitor your portions. Your mid-morning snack should contain no more than 150–250 calories or about 15 percent of your total daily calories.

Lunch

Lunch is essential for everyone every day, but it's especially crucial if you plan to exercise in the afternoon. Ideally, you want to eat complex carbohydrates, especially if your activity requires endurance. Marlia advises you to look at your plate: Normally, 50 percent or more of the calories should be from carbohydrates; when you are training, you should bump that up to 60 percent carbohydrates. Carbs are not just bagels, rice, and bread—carbs are also fruits, vegetables, beans, and milk.

A salad with corn or potatoes is a good choice. In Europe, we add anchovies; apparently, no one in the United States likes anchovies, but you can add a hard-boiled egg (the white only), capers, tomatoes, and a spoonful of oil, a little salt, and vinegar if you like vinegar. You could have a slice of bread with the salad, but the vegetables and corn also impart carbohydrates.

You want to eat some protein at lunch, too, for its satiating qualities and to slow the absorption of carbohydrates into your bloodstream. Protein plays an important role in growth, repair, and maintenance of muscle, and in supporting your immune system. Good protein sources include lean animal products (such as beef, chicken, fish, eggs, and milk), as well as soy, nuts, whole grains, and beans. Nutritious lunches include:

■ A low-fat bean burrito and green salad
■ A green salad with beans and tuna canned in water
■ A turkey sandwich on whole wheat bread with fruit
■ Low-fat cottage cheese with vegetables and a slice of whole grain bread

Be sure to drink another two to three eight-ounce glasses of water with lunch to start your afternoon well hydrated.

Afternoon and Pre-Training Snacks

The time between lunch and dinner can be upward of six to eight hours, which is *a long* time to go without eating. An afternoon snack is critical to helping you get through the second half of your busy day and avoid coming home feeling ravenous. Your afternoon snack can vary depending on your plans. If you have a rest day and do not plan any fitness training, then your afternoon snack can be similar in content to your morning snack: include two food groups, 150 to 250 calories, and as much color as possible.

If you suffer from afternoon fatigue, Marlia suggests you look at your fluid intake for the day. When dehydrated, people often confuse thirst with hunger and eat something in response. However, you may not be experiencing low blood sugar but misinterpreting the signals as dehydration. By drinking some extra fluid in the afternoon, you reduce the number of calories you end up consuming for a snack, and you improve your mental status for that afternoon board meeting or making dinner with the kids.

If you plan to work out later in the day, you need to snack differently. Our recommendations for pre-training snacks will be covered later in the chapter.

Evening Meal

Though the last meal of the day is often shared with family and friends and is traditionally the biggest meal of the day, Marlia recommends you eat most of your calories during the early part of the day to fuel your activities rather than your sleep.

At the evening meal, include carbohydrates to restock your glycogen stores and protein to supply the hormones you release while you sleep to build and repair tissues. Especially when you're exercising, it's vital that you supply yourself with these essential building blocks at dinnertime.

By building blocks, however, we don't mean to imply that your servings should be brick-sized. Quite the contrary. If you divide your plate in quarters, two-quarters should be dedicated to vegetables, one-quarter to lean protein, and one-quarter to carbohydrates. Your carbs should be whole grain and roughly a half to one cup in size.

A serving of protein for the average adult is about the size of a deck of cards—about three ounces of meat. Most chicken breasts sold in grocery stores and served in restaurants are now around seven ounces—more than two servings. So be vigilant about the serving size (and its attendant calories).

Also, be aware that protein is the Trojan horse of eating for fitness. It's a great gift when you are working out and building lean body mass, but hidden inside many sources of protein you'll find the highest amount of fat of any food.

If you eat meat, choosing lower-fat cuts are your best defense. Choose:

- Chicken or turkey breast over thighs
- Pork tenderloin over pork chop
- Top sirloin over filet mignon

Always trim off as much visible fat as possible (this is saturated fat, the worst kind you can put in your body). If you suffer from high cholesterol, keep your meat consumption low.

We also advocate varying your protein sources. Eat:

- Fish two to three times a week (salmon, bass, tuna, halibut)
- Lean meat two to three times a week
- A vegetarian dish two to three times a week

Workout Fuel Prescription

Starting a new fitness program can be exhausting in itself, but to attempt physical activity with low energy can make exercising miserable. And this means you will be less inclined to go out and do it again tomorrow. We have put together what we consider the best timing and contents for food and fluid to boost your energy levels, make the most of your training time, and to fortify your recovery so you see maximum improvement and are braced for the next exercise session.

Before Exercise

The timing and the nutritional makeup of what you eat before exercising matters. If you exercise in the morning or evening, your afternoon snack should follow two to three hours after your lunch. If you exercise in the afternoon—say, directly after you get off work, for example—your afternoon snack should be timed with regard to your workout. We typically recommend the afternoon snack (and two eight-ounce cups of water) two to four hours before exercise.

The size and composition of the snack or meal depends on the amount of time between when you eat it and when you will start to exercise. The more time you have, the larger the meal should be; the less time, the smaller the meal and the less protein and fat it should contain.

Food Three Hours Before a Workout

Lunch three hours before a 3 p.m. bike ride could include a turkey sandwich with avocado, a piece of fruit, and a cup of yogurt. A meal such as this, containing fat and protein, slows down digestion and the absorption of carbohydrates, which means you maintain more level blood sugar over time. This is particularly important when your workout occurs three hours later.

Food One Hour Before a Workout

For an early morning run, have a small snack (such as half an energy bar or a piece of fruit) thirty minutes to an hour before. When eating an hour or closer to the time you'll exercise, choose foods that are easily digestible and absorbable so the carbohydrates will be available for use by your body during your workout. If you consumed this same snack three hours before exercise, however, you would feel hungry and might experience low blood sugar at the beginning of your workout.

The principle at work here regarding blood sugar is called the glycemic index mentioned earlier. The glycemic index of a food is measured by how rapidly it increases your blood sugar. Carbohydrate-based foods have a high or low glycemic index. Those carbohydrates that contain more complex carbohydrates and fiber (whole grains, beans, and vegetables) typically have a low glycemic index. This means the food gradually increases your blood sugar and then levels off over time. Foods that contain simple carbohydrates (milk, yogurt, honey, fruit, and products with high-fructose corn syrup) have a high glycemic index. This means you rapidly digest and absorb the carbohydrates, which raises your blood sugar immediately. And, as you know, what goes up must come down. Your blood sugar then crashes thirty to forty-five minutes later.

The glycemic index of a carbohydrate is influenced by fat and protein that is eaten with it. Take, for example, a high glycemic index food such as fruit and add a tablespoon of peanut butter. The fat and protein in peanut butter slow down digestion and absorption of the fruit's carbohydrates, changing your overall blood sugar response to the fruit.

Ultimately, we dissuade athletes from eating any high-glycemic foods as close as a half hour before exercising, especially if they plan to do an endurance workout. The ensuing blood sugar crash will guarantee that you'll hit the wall about forty-five minutes into your workout. Instead, we favor a low-glycemic snack an hour and a half before you exercise.

Fuel During Exercise

If your workout is shorter than an hour and low intensity, during your workout you likely need to consume water only. If you're doing high-intensity intervals (hill repeats as a cyclist, for example, or sprints if you're running), or if your workout spans more than an hour to an hour and a half, you will need carbohydrates as well as water. The American College of Sports Medicine recommends eating and drinking during such exercise. The recommendations include drinking five to eleven fluid ounces of fluid every fifteen–twenty minutes and eating 30–60 grams of carbohydrates every hour during exercise that lasts longer than one hour. Carbohydrates help support your blood sugar, which supplies your brain and working muscles during exercise when your glycogen stores start to run low. Vary your carbohydrate sources. Good options include:

- Sports drinks
- Gels
- Fruit
- Fig bars
- Energy bars
- Whole wheat crackers
- Pretzels
- Dried fruit

Your mid-exercise snacks should be predominately carbohydrates with a little protein and fat. Check the label: You're aiming for 25–50 grams of carbohydrates, fewer than 5 grams of protein, and fewer than 3 grams of fat per serving.

People who do not fuel themselves during longer workouts often fail to get the maximum benefit from their workout. If they had only eaten some carbs during that precious hour and a half of exercise they squeezed into their busy lives, they may have lifted five more pounds, increased their power output, or gone faster. Ideally, start eating thirty minutes into your training session. Don't wait until you are hungry because by then your blood sugar level has already dropped and your performance has already suffered.

People often assume that eating during training is not wise if you're aiming to lose weight, but we're not talking about eating a Subway sandwich while at the gym for two hours. Bring along something low in calories and high in carbohydrates. People who don't fuel while they are working out not only lose out on a quality workout, but they often feel ravenous afterward, which leads to overeating and storing more of the calories they consume as fat.

To take full advantage of carbohydrate absorption, you need about eight ounces of water to every 14 grams of carbohydrates (that comes out to a drink that is about 6–8 percent carbohydrates). Be aware of combining a carbohydrate drink with a high-carbohydrate snack during exercise. For example, if you add a Gu pack—25 grams of carbohydrates—to the 14 grams of carbohydrates mixed into your water, you might slow down absorption. Very sensitive people could even experience cramping or vomiting. In any case, it will slow your body's ability to absorb either the carbohydrates or the water and you will not get them into your bloodstream as quickly as you had hoped. This again will lower how vigorously you are able to exercise.

To gauge whether or not you consumed enough calories during exercise, you should not feel starving when you finish.

Recovery Prescription

Following a high-intensity workout or one that's an hour to an hour and a half in length, you need to eat some carbohydrates to help replenish your glycogen stores. You have a window of fifteen to thirty minutes after exercise when your body tends to absorb and your muscles tend to better utilize whatever you give them. This is the ideal time to consume carbohydrates because immediately after you finish exercising your body changes enzyme activity, setting the stage to refuel your glycogen stores in your muscles and your liver in preparation for the next bout of exercise. A perfect high-intensity recovery snack contains 25 to 30 grams of carbohydrates. Good choices include:

- Half an energy bar
- Sixteen fluid ounces of an energy drink

It's imperative that you concentrate on carbohydrates at this time because your body is very inclined to store it for future exercise. It's also worthwhile replenishing your stores for the purpose of supplying your mental performance and any other activity you need to do later in the day. A busy mom who needs to drive the kids to soccer practice after exercising won't be tired and depleted of energy. If you go back to work after your workout, you will be able to concentrate better. If you go for a second workout or engage in other physical activity later, you'll be ready to go. All of these hinge, however, on your having restocked your energy pantry within that thirty-minute post-exercise window. Proper post-exercise eating will also improve your recovery, Marlia points out, and will prompt your desire to work out again.

A great way to get glucose calories fast is from a drink—it gets into your system much faster than food.

—Max

Finally, consume carbs and protein again two hours later, at a ratio of one gram of carbs and a half gram of protein per two pounds of body weight (so 80 grams of carbs and 40 of protein for someone who weighs 160 pounds). This could be a regular meal.

This will continue your glycogen replenishment and the recovery and rebuilding of your muscle tissue.

Recovery Hydration

Don't forget fluids. Drink at least sixteen fluid ounces after any type of exercise.

Weigh yourself before and after exercise. Any weight you have lost is *fluid loss* and needs to be replaced for adequate recovery. Your goal is to maintain your pre-exercise weight. For every pound you've lost during exercise, drink sixteen fluid ounces (one pint) afterward. And next time you exercise, drink more fluid than you did this time.

After strength-training exercise, have a recovery drink that contains branch-chain amino acids (to make up proteins), especially valine, leucine, and isoleucine. It should also have carbs, which tell your muscles to use the protein.

If you consume a recovery drink, be sure you drink it during the fifteen- to thirty-minute window. Studies show that the best recovery drinks contain protein and carbs. Modulate these depending on what you do.

Carbohydrates Are Quintessential

It's pretty clear now why carbohydrates are the best calories to consume as you embark on any exercise program. Your carbohydrate stores are your tank of gas. If you allow your tank of gas to run near empty most of the time, you're basically sputtering through your day, and may run out of gas when you try to gun it during exercise. You won't make it over the hill or, if you do, you'll be miserable trying. Your brain lives off carbohydrates exclusively, which means that your carbohydrate intake influences your performance not only during exercise but in school, at work, and in social situations. You are what you eat, yes, but you are primarily *the carbohydrates* that you eat.

Weight-Loss Pitfalls

In our experience, people who really struggle with getting fit and losing weight share an exquisite thing in common. Or rather, they share the lack of one thing.

Time.

Many of us are squeezing every moment from our days already. In her work, Marlia finds that it's very common for people to feel tired during exercise while also struggling to lose weight because they have a very busy schedule. To get fit, some of that time you commit to fitness should be spent on guaranteeing that you eat well. Planning meals and snacks is usually last on the list of priorities because food seems so accessible. If you forget to pack a nutritious lunch, you can easily walk out of your office door and either hit the break room or run across the street to the deli.

Ask yourself how often you eat out. People forget how often they go out and how much they eat when they do. Going out for dinner is probably on your radar, but how many times a week do you eat breakfast or lunch out? Often people forget about those muffins they grab with coffee on the way to work, or those spur-of-the-moment lunches with coworkers. When people keep track for a week, some discover they eat out as much as twice or more a day. Again, time is the culprit: They didn't have time to eat breakfast at home, they didn't have time to shop for or pack a lunch.

Eating out is costly in terms of calories. Even what might appear to be healthy choices at restaurants may have loads of additional calories. You might get sucked into salads with candied nuts, too much dressing, and several ounces of cheese. Some salads have the same number of calories as a hamburger and fries.

First count the number of times you eat out per week so you become conscious of the frequency. Then minimize eating out any meals or snacks to no more than a couple of times per week. For some people that's not possible because they have to go to business lunches or entertain clients. For others, it's a matter of preparedness: They need to learn how to shop for food to have on hand.

Of course time, again, is of the essence. People have all sorts of time constraints centered on eating at home: They don't have time for the shopping, the preparation, or the cleanup.

Marlia recommends several techniques for getting over the very real time hurdles. First, *do* grocery shop, even if you can't go frequently. When healthy food is just a refrigerator or a lunch bag away, it is in fact *faster* than fast food. And you'll save calories and money, and eat better, too. Here are some guidelines:

Shopping Strategies

- Shop the perimeter of the store—that's where you will find the least processed foods. Avoid the aisles; they primarily contain empty calories, according to Braun.
- Buy fresh fruits and vegetables to consume over the next two to three days.

- Choose smaller, single-serving size apples, bananas, and other fruit rather than the super-sized ones often available. This will help keep your portion size down.
- Get over any fears of frozen. Frozen vegetables are a healthy option; are also easy to keep around; and come prewashed, trimmed, and cut up for quick preparation. They work particularly well in stir-fries, soups, and with pasta and grains.
- Marlia also recommends stockpiling whole-grain pastas and other kinds of grains to cook up on the fly. "Throw in some frozen vegetables and you've got a meal—and only one pan to wash."
- Canned vegetables are higher in sodium and contain less fiber, nutrients, and phytochemicals than fresh vegetables, but they're still better than eating a candy bar.
- Fruits canned in their own juices (not syrup) and drained are another option.
- Check out the frozen prepacked meals. Low-calorie, low-sodium options such as Healthy Choice, Weight Watchers, and Smart Ones are good sources of fiber and protein, don't go over 180 to 300 calories, are well balanced, and they always provide a portion of protein and a grain.
- Think variety. Your goal on any grocery shopping venture is a colorful grocery bag; this ensures you'll be adding a wide range of fruits and vegetables. Each hue offers different nutrients, and it's important to include some of each every week. Instead of buying a large quantity of one thing (say, seven oranges for breakfast for the next week), buy a peach or strawberries for one day, a mango or banana for the next, and so on.
- Ditto for vegetables: Don't plan to eat red bell peppers or spinach at every meal. Plan a different veggie for each meal each day. Variety is fundamental to the longevity and sustainability of a diet as well as to getting adequate nutrients for your hardworking body.
- Mix your whole grains. Try barley and quinoa as well as brown rice and whole wheat. At least half of your carbohydrates should be whole grains. Look for "100 percent whole grain" on the package. It should also be listed as the first ingredient.
- Each week, sample fruits or vegetables you don't normally buy. Try cauliflower instead of broccoli, edamame instead of peas. Simmer Brussels sprouts in chicken soup (delicious!) or make a red cabbage slaw instead of your usual spring mix salad.
- Go shopping or cook with friends to see the healthy, low-fat foods they

prepare. Try the Internet for ideas on how to prepare new low-fat meals.

- Don't abstain from foods you love. You can keep your favorite foods, just reduce your portions and frequency. For example, have one ounce of chocolate twice a week rather than a bar every day.

Here are more of Marlia's shopping tips:

GROCERY SHOPPING 101
Healthy Performance Food Choices for People Who Can't Shop Often

Produce section

Fruit that stays fresh for more than a week	**More perishable**
apples	bananas, grapes
oranges, tangerines	berries, kiwi
melons, grapefruit	pears, peaches, plums

Vegetables that are longer lasting	**More perishable**
carrots, celery, zucchini, squash	broccoli, cucumbers
sweet and white potatoes, yams	tomatoes, mushrooms
red or green cabbage, onions	fresh spinach, sprouts
cauliflower, Brussels sprouts	dark green leafy lettuces
green beans, peas	
artichoke, asparagus	

Meats, fish, eggs and meat alternatives

Ground turkey 98% fat free, ground beef 98% fat free, luncheon meats, pre-cut pieces of chicken, pork, beef, fish fillets, shellfish, eggs or egg substitute, baked/flavored tofu

Frozen foods

Berries, melon, peaches

Corn, peas, peas and carrots, pearl onions, variety mixes, spinach

Chicken breasts, fish fillets, shellfish, burritos, stir-fry mixes, garden burgers, veggie burgers

Dairy Case

Low-fat or fat-free yogurt or soy yogurt

Low-fat cheese or soy cheese

Low-fat cottage cheese

Skim milk

Low-fat soy milk

Pantry items

Whole-grain cereals, instant oatmeal

Whole-grain bread, bagels, tortillas, pitas, pasta, couscous

Wild and brown rice

Beans, canned (kidney, garbanzo, black)

Soups (broth with chicken and vegetables), chili

Fruit, canned in lite syrup or own juice (peaches, pineapple, mixed fruit)

Vegetables, canned (green beans, corn, tomatoes, tomato paste)

Canned tuna, salmon, chicken packed in water

Powdered nonfat milk

Old-fashioned peanut butter, almond butter, lite jams or preserves

Courtesy of Marlia Braun, Ph.D., R.D., UC Davis Sports Medicine

Strategies for Eating Out

If you are prone to eat out often or overindulge when you do eat out, we advocate the following strategies:

- When you go out to eat, you may feel you can order everything: drinks, appetizers, wine with your meal, dessert. That's more than you would eat at home, and certainly more than you need to consume at one sitting. Instead, be mindful of what you order when you do eat out and limit it.
- Look at the menu, giving priority to low-fat, nutrient-dense options.
- Find dishes, plates, or entrées that keep the food groups separate; one-dish meals often have too much added fat from oil, butter, and cheese, making it hard to estimate the calories. A piece of grilled fish, steamed veggies, and a side of grains have a limited amount of fat.
- When ordering veggies, ask to have them steamed rather than sautéed.
- If the meal comes with mashed potatoes, ask for a baked potato instead and limit the condiments.
- Ask the cook to sideline the sauces and dressings.
- Like at home, trim visible fat off meats.

Here are good fast-food options:

BEST CHOICES FOR EATING OUT

Fast Food	Calories	Fat (gm)	Carbs (gm)
McDonald's			
BBQ Chicken Sandwich	340	8	48
Chicken Fajita Roll-up	190	7	21
Chicken McGrill (w/o mayo)	280	16	34
Whole Wheat Grilled Chicken	320	7	39
Hamburger	280	10	36
McVeggie Burger w/ cheese	405	12	47
Grilled Chicken California Cobb	265	11	9
Grilled Chicken Bacon Ranch Salad	250	10	9
Fruit'n Yogurt Parfait w/ granola	155	2	30
Taco Bell			
Bean Burrito	370	10	55
Fiesta Burrito Chicken	370	13	48
Regular Taco	170	10	13
Soft Taco Chicken	190	6	19
Soft Taco Supreme Chicken	230	10	21
Gordita Nacho Cheese, Chicken or Steak	290	10	30
Pintos and cheese	180	7	20
Tostada	250	10	29
Togo's			
Farmer's Market (9 oz)	120	3	18
Oriental Salad (21.3 oz)	390	7	53
Black Bean Soup	200	7	27
Chicken Noodle Soup	150	3.5	20
New England Clam Chowder	105	6	6
Albacore Tuna Sandwich (reg.)	455	10	69
Turkey and Cheese (reg.)	600	18	71
Carl's Jr.			
Charboiled Chicken Sandwich	365	4	47
Hamburger	280	9	38
Potato, plain	280	0	63

Other options	Calories	Fat (gm)	Carbs (gm)
Applebee's (low-fat menu)			
Asian Chicken Salad	715	9	121
Blackened Chicken Salad	425	8.5	39
Chicken Fajita Quesadilla	520	11	63

Chicken Rancho Rollup	590	12	80
Chicken Roma Rollup	640	10	83
Chicken Pasta	530	11	78
Garlic-Lemon Chicken Pasta	530	11	78
Veggie Quesadilla	595	12	86
Whitefish w/ Mango Salsa	435	10	54
Chili's			
Chicken Grill Pita	545	9	77
Chicken Platter	565	9	83
Chicken Sandwich	525	8	70
Citrus Fire Chicken & Shrimp	660	12	73
Hawaiian Steak	685	13	88
Ginger Citrus Glazed Salmon	710	22	70
Chicken Caesar Pita (no fries)	520	19	33
Olive Garden			
Capellini Pomodora (13 oz)	350	11	52
Chicken Giardino (15.5 oz)	350	7	40
Linguine alla Marinara (10.6 oz)	280	6	48
Shrimp Primavera (19 oz)	490	15	65
Denny's			
Chicken Noodle Soup (8 oz)	60	2	8
Vegetable Beef (8 oz)	80	1	11
Grilled Chicken S'wich (w/o dressing)	495	14	56
Turkey Breast on Multigrain	290	4	41
Fried Shrimp Dinner	230	10	18
Grilled Chicken Dinner	205	5	15
Pot Roast Dinner w/Gravy	290	11	5
Roast Turkey & Stuffing w/Gravy	505	10	62
Grilled Chicken Breast Salad	230	11	10
Garden Deluxe Salad w/ Chicken	230	11	10
Side Garden Salad, w/o dressing	115	4	16

Courtesy of Marlia Braun, Ph.D., R.D., UC Davis Sports Medicine

Other Weight-Loss Pitfalls

Many people get discouraged because they believe that starting to exercise invariably causes weight loss. Unfortunately, not always. We encounter many people who finally decide to exercise, and then gain weight. Understanding why this happens may help.

Many people celebrate their new quest for fitness by overrewarding themselves with a beer they would not have otherwise had, or by eating more. And, yes, they gain weight. Avoid this mistake, eat fewer calories than you burn, and you will lose weight.

A premenopausal woman or a man in his early fifties can gain fifteen to twenty pounds quite suddenly, in about a year, even though they are exercising and have not changed their diet.

For these people to lose weight, Marlia suggests they eliminate hidden and empty calories such as cocktails and wine, which people often over-look and underestimate. (Consuming alcohol is also dehydrating, which can impact the quality of your workouts.) A glass of wine contains about 100 calories, a beer or vodka tonic 150, a small margarita 185 (the fishbowl variety can contain up to 1,000 calories), and creamy specialty drinks, particularly those containing coconut milk, pack about 350 calories.

Avoid the "Entitlement Meal"

Your after-workout meal should not be an engorgement. In fact, this is why many people fail to lose weight when they begin to exercise: the devi-ous "entitlement meal." Ever had one? This meal consists of everything you want, because you deserve it. You're working out, you feel entitled. But this will negate your weight-loss efforts.

Change It Up

Vary the exercise you do. If you get too comfortable with your workout and don't challenge yourself, your body will stop adapting or improving because it no longer perceives the exercise as overload. And you won't see the progress you were hoping for.

To get a jump-start on your weight loss safely without compromising the quality of your food intake, see Max's Jumpstart Weight-Loss Diet on page 103.

WEATHERING WORKOUTS

Heating Up!

A hot environment is one of the most severe stresses an athlete can en-dure. Just like a car, you need water to cool your engine. When you exer-cise, your muscle contractions cause heat. Every machine needs energy to produce work and that energy produces heat. Even in the best man-made machine, only about 20 to 25 percent of the energy goes to work and 75 percent goes to heat.

Without enough water, the heat produced by activity puts you at risk for injury in hot weather. Your organs and the chemical reactions within your body work only within a precise range of temperature and acidity. If you go outside this ideal range, you become hypothermic (too cold) or hyperthermic (too hot). An increase in core temperature can cause cardiac problems, for example. Thus, keeping your body temperature constant is a high priority for your body.

One factor you need to be aware of is the ambient air temperature. When air temperatures exceed your skin temperature, your body's ability to release heat is compromised. Another factor that you need to consider is humidity. When you perspire, sweat evaporates from your skin, which brings your temperature down. High humidity prevents evaporation. When your sweat drips off of you, it's no longer evaporating, and that means it's no longer cooling your body. In both cases, you'll need to manage the additional heat.

To keep your body temperature constant, drinking water is a must. You will hit the wall very quickly if you are not drinking. Water has a high thermal capacity so it's able to keep your temperature constant. In fact, drinking water before, during, and after exercise is *more* important than fuel. In hot conditions, you can lose anywhere from two to three liters of fluid per hour. If you do not replace the lost fluid, your volume of circulating blood will decrease, making your heart pump faster, which can result in fatigue and possibly death.

Thus, you need to be well hydrated for exercise. To keep up with fluid losses and manage heat, Marlia recommends that you:

- Plan for frequent fluid breaks during exercise.
- Avoid caffeinated, alcoholic, and carbonated beverages, which can enhance your dehydration or result in less fluid consumed.
- Replenish your electrolytes, in particular sodium, to avoid hyponatremia, or overhydration, during training and to optimize fluid retention post-training.

In addition, we also tell patients to:

- Check your weight before exercise.
- Drink a couple of glasses of water before exercise.
- Drink another eight to twelve ounces every fifteen to twenty minutes (half a liter to a full liter per hour) in hot weather.

- For very long-lasting activity, drink a little less (to avoid hyponatremia over the course of time).
- Two or three hours after the start of exercise, recheck your weight, and try to recover whatever weight you have lost in water. Remember the old cooking adage: "A pint's a pound the whole world 'round." In other words, for every pound you lose during exercise, you need to replace it by drinking a pint of water.

Three to four pounds is the maximum acceptable amount of water to lose. If you lose more than three or four pounds during an exercise session, in the future you need to:

- Drink more water beforehand
- Drink water several times before you head out (but never more than two pints at a time, or it will just sit in your stomach) *or*
- Drink more during exercise

Marlia recommends sports drinks over water because they are formulated to supply electrolytes as well as the ideal ratio of fluid to carbohydrates (they typically range from 6 to 8 percent carbohydrate). This is the perfect ratio for your stomach to absorb both, and thus provides immediate energy and fluid. Also, studies show that people who drink sports drinks during exercise consume more fluid on average compared to people who drink plain water.

If you continue to sweat for a half hour after exercise, this is a sign that your body is still trying to lower your core temperature, which means you became overheated and need to be more careful next time.

For gym workouts during extreme weather, you do not need to consume as much water because you're not sweating as much, but you still need to consume some water. Add carbohydrates if your workout is going to last over one hour.

Brrr!

The most common problem training in cold environments is hypothermia. During cold training sessions, your body needs to provide not only the energy for training but also the energy for maintaining your body's core temperature. This is even costlier if you are training at altitude.

When your body loses heat faster than you can produce it, your body will cool. This restricts blood flow to your working muscles, which translates to a workout lower in quality and quantity.

If you are training in the cold weather, Marlia recommends you drink fluids often. This is important to remember since cold exposure can reduce your sense of hunger and thirst. When exercising in the cold, hydration is also important. In cold weather:

- Drink 8 to 12 ounces every hour.
- Have a sports drink, in order to consume carbs with your water. Choose whatever variety you like the best, then you will be sure to drink it (which is not always easy to do in the cold).
- If you do a two-hour workout in cold temperatures, use a drink that is 6 to 8 percent carbohydrate, the upper range of carb-to-water ratio for good absorption.
- You need not be as concerned about the sodium content of the drink in cold weather as you would in heat.

She also notes that the combination of cold temperatures and exercise does not necessarily boost your fat metabolism. In fact, your fat metabolism may be lower when exercising in the cold, possibly due to the vasoconstriction of peripheral fat tissue.

However, you may also benefit from a few extra calories to avoid weight loss due to the extra energy expenditure in maintaining your body temperature. Adding more nutrient-dense high-carbohydrate foods such as trail mix with nuts or freeze-dried foods can help you support energy needs when training in the cold.

Supplements

No discussion of exercise and nutrition would be complete without addressing the question of supplements. If you simply went on the information given by the companies that make and sell vitamins and other supplements, you might think that a cupboard full are necessary once you begin exercising. Not true.

> When I was training for and competing in the Olympics, and as a pro cyclist, and as I weight-trained all my life, the only supplement I took was one multivitamin a day. That's it.
>
> —Eric

Many people who seek fitness who are also cutting back their caloric intake to fewer than 1,600 per day should consider a simple multivitamin and multimineral supplement. When consuming low calories, it can be difficult to meet all of your vitamin and mineral needs.

When looking for a multivitamin multimineral supplement, find one by a company that makes lots of different supplements. This can help assure a higher-quality product even though supplements are not currently regulated by the Food and Drug Administration (FDA). Also, look for one that contains around 100 percent of the U.S. Recommended Dietary Allowance. The purpose of the multivitamin and multimineral is to complement what you have already consumed via your diet. These supplements are not meant to substitute for a poor diet. Also, keep in mind that your vitamin and mineral recommendations are meant to be met over several days, not necessarily every day.

Avoid supplements that are labeled "mega" doses. Many vitamins and minerals are toxic at high levels and even when nontoxic they can interfere with the normal metabolism of other minerals. Keep in mind, many foods are now fortified with extra vitamins and minerals. In fact, many sports bars and cereals can substitute for a multivitamin and multimineral pill. If you eat these regularly, you may not need a separate vitamin-mineral supplement.

Getting your vitamins and minerals from foods is far more beneficial than getting them from a pill. Nutrients in foods assist the absorption and utilization of other nutrients. For the same reason, take your supplement with food and fluids to encourage proper absorption and utilization.

What if I'm a schoolteacher. How can I possibly eat five meals a day?

We know that even a teacher's "breaks" are filled with obligations. Between classes, during recess, when the kids have their snack time, make having a couple of carrots or an apple part of what you have to do during that break.

In addition, many school districts have no prohibition about teachers munching a celery stick in class—check with yours. It certainly won't harm kids to see their teacher having a healthy mid-afternoon snack, and it's critical for your health. Consider it a medical prescription.

What if I keep my eating in check all day, but I'm ravenous at night?

It's possible that you are not eating enough during the day. Remember, fuel your day and not your sleep. Try adding a healthy snack or increasing your portions to avoid a large evening meal or evening bingeing.

What if after a serious workout I get hungry?

To prepare for the demands of a hard workout, two to four hours beforehand have a meal or snack with a good source of carbohydrate, and consume 30–60 grams of carbohydrate every hour while you work out. Last, stave off fatigue by being well hydrated. Drink sixteen fluid ounces one to two hours before and five to eleven fluid ounces for every twenty minutes of exercise. Start drinking and eating early. Avoid having to respond to hunger and thirst. Keep ahead of them.

What if I never have time to cook a good meal after I get home from work, the gym, the PTA meeting . . . ?

Max's wife, Julie: Boil pasta. Sauté garlic in a little olive oil, then add chopped fresh vegetables. Drain the pasta, then toss it with the sautéed mixture. *Fifteen* minutes!

Max: Better idea: Boil pasta, and throw in fresh broccoli while the pasta is boiling, drain, then garnish with a little olive oil and Parmesan. *Ten* minutes!

Eric: Even better: Take a slice of bread, spread on peanut butter, then sprinkle on chopped raw onion. *Two* minutes!

Max's Jump-Start Weight-Loss Diet

Everyone wants to lose weight when they get fit, and success with weight at the start is very motivating. The problem with many diets that promise immediate short-term success is that they are unbalanced and simply cause weight loss through dehydration or muscle loss. I have a diet that I've been using for fifteen years that helps my athletes lose weight without dehydration or muscle loss.

Normally, I propose this diet to my patients for two weeks just to give them a boost for weight loss. When that happens, and they lose five or six pounds, and start to feel their pants are a little loose at the waist, and they have to punch a new hole in their belt, they get *very* motivated. They can feel their stomach sucking in maybe for the first time in a while and they feel good. It is worthwhile to have quick, visible improvement in the first two weeks as a source of motivation. The diet consists of 1,600–1,800 calories. It doesn't matter where they are when they start, if they eat like this for two weeks, they all lose at least three or four pounds.

Please note: This is a starter diet for healthy people (those who have checked with their doctor and have no medical problems). It is also intended for very short-term use only—no longer than two weeks.

BREAKFAST

The day starts with a half liter of tea—the equivalent of two or three normal cups of tea. You can add one spoon of honey and skim milk, if you like. You sip that for the first hour after you get up.

MID-MORNING SNACK

Around mid-morning, eat two servings of fruit. I favor one banana along with an apple, a pear, a handful of strawberries, a peach, or a plum. Vary the fruit you eat each day with your banana. Drink two glasses of water beforehand.

LUNCH

At midday, I suggest another piece of fruit and a sandwich with whole wheat bread. It can be turkey or ham and cheese, or plain tuna, with tomato and lettuce, but no mayonnaise, no mustard. Drink another two glasses of water beforehand.

MID-AFTERNOON SNACK AND/OR BEFORE EXERCISE

Have a protein bar in the middle of the afternoon, along with another two glasses of water. I encourage eating a bar or another carbohydrate snack buffered with protein before exercise because to get the full benefit of exercising you don't want to get hungry and hit the wall during training.

DINNER

For your evening meal, eat salad, a serving of fruit or vegetables, and a serving of fish or meat. No bread. And, again, water.

I have never known anyone who did this for two weeks and did not lose weight. This is by no means a diet that one should continue long-term, but for a short time it's not harmful.

"My grandmother started walking five miles a day when she was sixty. She's ninety-three now and we don't know where the hell she is."

—ELLEN DeGENERES

6

better progress

In preparation for the Olympics, ancient Greeks lifted the same calf daily, and the amount of weight they could lift increased as the calf grew. This, in essence, is the famed exercise scheduling technique known as progressive overload. It's an easy concept to understand. It has just one fault: It doesn't always work.

Modern fitness-seekers, too, follow this ancient-style, popularized form of improvement and work themselves into the ground, then give up their fitness program due simply to fatigue. Take, for example, the most popular (and magical) method of periodization. Want to run a marathon, twenty-six miles? Just run a mile today, add a mile tomorrow, a third the third day, and in twenty-six days, you will be able to run twenty-six miles, right? Ditto for weight lifting or cycling. Just add a little more every day until you reach your goal. What could be simpler? In reality, after very few days even an athlete with nearly infinite promise is unable to add more. So she misses a day or two. Or, worse, she forges ahead and does herself harm. Then, if she's like most people, she'll view her fitness effort as a failure and believe she is not meant to exercise.

There are several forms of periodization that work, but the version that has been sold to fitness-seekers—and ancient Greeks—is oversimplified. Biologically sound methods of periodization reinforce a regular fitness habit. People learn to anticipate fatigue and plan for it. When they're fatigued, instead of skipping a day or giving up altogether, they simply exercise muscles or systems that are fresh, and allow time for the fatigued systems of their body to recover.

Everyone develops adaptations at a different rate. At the beginning of my career I worked with bodybuilders. I observed that when they did the same number of repetitions, lifting the same weight, they developed at different rates. And with bodybuilders, those who don't get big, get mad.

—Max

As you exercise, don't expect daily swells in your ability. Your biologic improvement will not be a linear progression, with a steady rise day after day. Numerous exercise programs chart perfect arcs representing the gradual increase in the amount of required exercise you should do, as if your body will continuously build at the same rate every day indefinitely. Instead, expect to get stronger in waves. One day you'll feel dormant, another day you will leaf out like you can't believe. That's due to the fact that any type of exercise training you do is actually working many systems in your body: your lungs, your heart, your muscles, and your energy delivery system. Each of these systems requires a different length of time to recover and repair, thus they bear gains at varying rates.

Your cardiovascular system, for example, delivers quickly. If you go running, you will feel cardiovascular fatigue immediately, even as you exercise: You will become out of breath, and you will know precisely when you are tired. You will also profit quickly. Within as little as two days you may see improved cardiovascular fitness: It will be easier to go farther, and your breathing will be less labored. However, you also lose cardiovascular fitness quickly. If you have years of aerobic exercise under your belt, the vast cardiovascular constructions you have repeatedly fortified won't be torn down by your body as quickly. But if you are new to exercise, within days after your last aerobic workout your brand-new improvements will be demolished and carted away.

At the other end of the spectrum, you will discover that some types of muscular training require substantial time before you feel fatigue, and substantial time to recover and repair. Muscle fatigue results from actual microscopic tears in your muscles, which can require time to heal to a point where the muscles can perform again. For instance, plyometrics (a type of strengthening using explosive movements, such as those done with a jump rope or on a trampoline) require a recovery as long as eleven days. With muscular strengthening the sense of fatigue also comes slowly. When you lift weights or do other weight-bearing exercise, you won't feel muscle fatigue at the time you exercise. You can do two sets of twelve repetitions and feel like you haven't done anything, but the next day your muscles feel sore. Because you don't feel fatigue while you have the weight in your hands, it's tempting to do more than your program advises, but that can cause injury or soreness that will keep you from exercising again anytime soon. So with muscular strengthening, don't depend on a sense of fatigue to dictate when to stop.

Somewhere on the spectrum, between the quick turnaround of aerobic payback and the ponderous pace of muscle compensation, lies the rate of recovery of your other biologic systems.

Because each system's recovery occurs at a different rate, the trick is to properly combine all the elements in a schedule where the fatigue of a single system never overwhelms your ability to exercise. However, this poses a bit of a conundrum. To flourish, you must challenge your body dramatically enough and frequently enough to send a clear, consistent message that you want it to accommodate more; however, you must also respect the time each system requires to recover, reinforce, and return, ready to take on more.

Enter periodization. Periodization sounds like a complicated concept, but you will use it to simplify your daily and monthly exercise schedule and to pace your exercise and your expectations. Effective forms of periodization interweave the three elements that are the daily bread of exercise: workout, fatigue, and recovery. Your schedule will tell you when to embrace more activity, when to hold back, and how to deal with normal fatigue. Essentially you will maximize your return on your exercise investment by planning to alternate hard and easy days, and hard and easy weeks, for each system of your body. These waves of activity are tied directly to the speed of fatigue, recovery, and improvement of each system.

Let's look at a hypothetical periodized exercise calendar:

Monday: Rest
Tuesday: Warm-up and run (biggest aerobic day)
Wednesday: Warm-up and muscle strengthening
Thursday: Warm-up, swim, bike, or yoga
Friday: Warm-up and run
Saturday: Warm-up, yoga or Pilates, and swim (optional)
Sunday: Warm-up and muscle strengthening
Start week again

This schedule anticipates that on Tuesday, at the beginning of your workout week, after rest on Monday you will feel aerobically fresh. That's the day you schedule your hardest aerobic workout. The next day your cardiovascular system will be spent, thanks to the work it did the day before, but your muscles will be ready to go. Thus, you will do muscle strengthening for your upper body. This way you allow your cardiovascular system (and your legs) to rest and recover, but you still make use of the day to challenge another part of your body. The third day you will want to give your upper-body muscles a break, but your lungs and heart rested the day before, so you will do another aerobic workout. On Thursday you will anticipate the fatigue from lifting the day before, and you will plan to give your legs a break with active recovery: yoga and swimming. You swim because your lungs and heart had a day off Wednesday, and you do core strengthening (via yoga or a Pilates class) because the muscles in your abdomen and back are fresh. Friday you do another aerobic workout. In this schedule, on muscle-strengthening days, you will do a twenty-minute warm-up run at a pleasant pace. On days when you go hard on muscular strengthening, you'll do only a light warm-up.

In this way, your exercise routine will be something of a puzzle: The pieces will fit together so that your body keeps progressing as some systems are stressed while others are recovering. Some days your muscles will feel very fatigued but your cardiovascular system will feel strong. On other days, you may feel your muscles are fresh, so you are able to push them in a great muscular-strengthening workout. Along the way, you will also dovetail in coordination and flexibility exercises. Following this pattern of repetition will allow your body to repair and build up the systems you worked the day (or days) before while using your exercise time to maximum profit.

Without understanding your biology, you might interpret the fatigue that occurs after any one of these days as a signal of weakness and the need to take a day off or to stop. But in fact this brand of fatigue, which halts many people in their tracks, is a positive signal and a necessary signpost along the road to becoming fit. You don't want to yield your goals when you feel the inevitable fatigue. Fatigue is a sign that you are right on the higher-voltage threshold.

For example, if you do muscle-strengthening exercise one day, and the next day you feel sore, many people might think: I did too much yesterday, I need to rest. But research shows that light exercise actually improves recovery from muscle-strengthening exercise. Someone who's educated on the process will manage muscle soreness in the proper way:

with low-impact exercise (an easy walk, bike ride, or swimming) and not waste the day on the couch.

After several weeks, your body will have adapted to handle the challenges of the progressive overload you've subjected it to, so you'll want to take it up a notch. Why? You know that lifting a pencil is not going to get you buffed; that's because it is not perceived by your body as overload. It's way below your ability. The same is true of a program you have been following for weeks or years. Your body now sees the workout as business as usual. It has long since risen to the occasion, so the workout doesn't place any new demands and doesn't trigger any new adaptations. When this happens, you plateau: You stop improving, stop losing weight, stop trimming seconds from your time. To continue to improve, you have to up the ante. We have several strategies for doing this and will discuss them later. At this point, suffice it to say that you are limited only by your potential.

PERIODIZATION IN ACTION

In the 1960s and 1970s, pioneering performance researcher Tudor Bompa, M.D., became baffled by something peculiar in the athletes he was studying. Less disciplined athletes who "called in well"—who essentially took days off from training—were doing better, by leaps and bounds, than the die-hard athletes who trained constantly. In fact, some of Dr. Bompa's most driven athletes, those who never took a day off, were suffering *reduced* performance.

It was a riddle wrapped in a mystery inside an enigma if he had ever seen one.

Dr. Bompa, already knee-deep in the dazzling complexities of how the human body develops, quickly ascertained that the secret to improving at an activity was to—now and then—*not* do it at all. He began experimenting with patterns of lighter, harder, and rest days, and then lighter, harder, and rest weeks. Slowly, he determined which patterns cultivated the highest rate of improvement.

Dr. Bompa went on to analyze what he'd unearthed and to describe it in training rules for maximum performance. From his work, four primary forms or modalities of periodization emerged, each based on one training month.

First Type of Periodization

Virtually anyone who has exercised has dabbled in the first type of periodization, whether he or she knows it or not. As we discussed at the beginning of the chapter, this form of periodization requires your body to improve at the same rate every day, day after day, indefinitely. So on New Year's Eve, if you decide you want to run the Western States 100 (a 100-mile trail run through the Rocky Mountains), you would run one mile on January 1, then two miles on January 2, and so on. And you would expect to be able to run 28 miles by January 28, and by mid-April you'd be all set to tackle the Western States 100.

Essentially this form of periodization dictates:

Week 1: Easy exercise
Week 2: Moderate exercise
Week 3: Harder exercise
Week 4: Hardest exercise
Repeat, with no recovery or rest weeks. Training load keeps increasing steadily month to month.

The flaw in this type of periodization is that if you exercise today, you aren't necessarily armed with the benefits tomorrow, or the next day—and in 100 days you will certainly not be able to run 100 miles. This example illustrates the point rather dramatically, but the same rule is true for small, incremental advancements as well. In the first two weeks, training won't be challenging enough for people who are fit; they lose two weeks. For people who are in bad shape, in the first two weeks their fatigue will develop faster than their improvements or adaptations; these people will get worse and worse day after day, not better and better.

Every day, your ability to train or perform is the difference between how fit you are from previous training minus your level of fatigue. You *are* getting better, but if you are becoming more fatigued faster, it overwhelms your fitness. We call this overreaching (which is different from overtraining, because you can recover in a few days). Effective training plays on the edge of how much you can recover and how much you can train. In reality this first type of periodization can fall over the edge.

Second Type of Periodization

This modality of periodization is used by most coaches we know. It allows your body to catch up after the hardest week of exercise.

Week 1: Easy exercise
Week 2: Moderate exercise
Week 3: Harder exercise
Week 4: Hardest exercise
Repeat. Exercise load does not necessarily escalate month to month (for example, Week 1 of the second month would not be harder than Week 4 of the first month).

This type of periodization doesn't take advantage of the fact that you are in the best condition when you are fresh after the first week. And the hardest week always falls when the athlete is already fatigued.

Third Type of Periodization

This form of periodization takes full advantage of the recovery week preceding the start of each cycle.

Week 1: Hardest exercise
Week 2: Hard exercise
Week 3: Moderate exercise
Week 4: Easiest exercise
Repeat.

This modality of periodization dictates the hardest week after the easiest week, which makes sense; you are in the best condition when you are fresh. The difficulty with the third type of periodization, however, is that even though the exercise in each successive week is "easier," it will feel harder due to the work you have done the previous week. Say, for example, you run 70 miles in the first and hardest week. In the second—supposedly easier—week, you run 55 to 65 miles, *but it will feel like 80.* During the third—and even easier—week, you run even fewer miles, but since it has been three weeks now since your last period of recovery, it is going to feel very difficult, and it will stretch your body tremendously. During the fourth week, you do active recovery, and will it be welcome! And when the cycle is repeated, the easiest/hardest weeks are in sync.

Some people will experience a huge leap in their performance when the cycle resumes with the first—and hardest—week again in the next cycle. For this reason, some athletes use this form of periodization to peak for a specific event. But it's important to know yourself; some people also find themselves overreaching. This is where training becomes more art than science. You have to know yourself and judge whether it works for you.

Fourth Type of Periodization

This modality works somewhat in reverse of the previous one. It's what we most often counsel people to use when they are in competition season.

Week 1: Hard exercise
Week 2: Easy week or tapering (details on tapering in Chapter 7, "Better Rest")
Week 3: Competition or hardest exercise
Week 4: Active rest*
Repeat.

The fourth type of periodization is successful because the hardest week is always followed by active rest, so recovery and adaptation are allowed to occur. Unlike the first type of periodization, the fourth modality doesn't place demands on your body that increase indefinitely. Instead, rest weeks are built in. (Our program also dictates rest days as an integral part of each week's schedule.)

> Skating, I used the second modality in the early phase, but when I wanted to have a big peak, I used the fourth mode.
>
> —Eric

Week to week in the program in Part Two, you will essentially plan the same sort of pattern, although the design gets a bit more sophisticated. You will alternate hard and easy sessions, by turns having days when you challenge your cardiovascular system and days when you challenge muscu-

---

*Active rest in this context means doing the same workouts but at a lower intensity and volume, or working on specific techniques you need to develop to avoid injury or improve your performance.

lar adaptation. Each of your systems will leapfrog ahead at its own pace while the system or systems you worked most recently are recovering, rebuilding, and preparing for their own leaps. While periodization in its strictest form will help you to prepare or peak for an event or a time period in the future when you want to be at your best, we are also applying it to your program on a day-by-day and week-to-week basis to capture your body's tiptop response. We do this by recommending exercise that alternates types and builds from easiest to hardest and then allows rest and recovery before building again. This form of periodization will help ensure your success.

The tempo of hard and easy days also changes as you gain fitness. In the beginning we will give you only one hard day followed by two easy days (totaling just two hard days each week) because in the beginning you are also training your ability to recover. Say you start with heavy days on Sunday and Thursday: At first it will take until Tuesday for you to feel recovered. However, in time you will feel recovered by Monday. When that happens, we will urge you to do three heavy days a week and then four, eventually progressing to two hard days back-to-back to stimulate even more improvements.

In our experience, when people realize that the march of improvement will not be steady, and they factor in fatigue and rest, over days and weeks, they learn how to pace their exercise *and* their expectations. And they succeed. Proper periodization makes improved fitness possible for everyone, and it doesn't stop after twelve weeks—it works for the rest of your life.

What if, on weekdays, I have an hour-long commute, I can't skip lunch to exercise because I eat breakfast early, and I can't exercise after work because I have to rush to pick up the kids, get groceries, make dinner, then help the kids with homework and baths and so on?

This is not ideal because in addition to infrequent exercise, you have a number of other stressors, which weigh on you physically. On weekends you can do only so much, and if you exercise just on weekends, you essentially have five days of rest, which is too long. Between one workout and the next, you almost completely lose any adaptations you gained.

If you can grab only one additional hour to exercise during your work-week (in addition to the exercise you get on the weekend), do that one hour midweek, and make it aerobic exercise. If you can find two hours to work out, spread them over two days, ideally a few days apart. And make the most of every exercise session you grab—no halfway efforts. Do the best you can every time you have a shot.

"Fatigue is the best pillow."

—Benjamin Franklin

7

better rest

Too busy or too tired to exercise? Many people come home from work, burned out and tired, but force themselves to exercise. And two hours later, they feel great: They are bursting with energy. They are able to sleep better. They are more productive. They can concentrate better. And they find they don't get as tired during the day on a regular basis. In fact, research reveals that sitting around may actually induce a greater sense of energy loss than exercise. Once people do take on exercise, however, they also need to factor in adequate rest, which, as you know, is an important element of your improvement plan.

The human race is increasingly workaholic, and it doesn't stop when it comes to exercise. Enthusiasm for exercise is fabulous. However, athletes who overdo it often get fatigued, sleep deprived, and overtrained (read: inadequate rest). Adequate rest is an important objective to attain. You may begin a fitness regimen and go at it like a fiend; then you get injured, ill, or too tired to continue—and you give up. The key is to follow your schedule and to understand the various kinds of rest you need as you exercise: rest days, tapering, and sleep.

If You Don't Snooze, You Lose

We encounter many people who are obsessive about every other area of their health but take for granted their body's daily requirement for sleep.

Sleep plays a significant role in your fitness. A lack of sufficient sleep can muffle your ability to exercise, to recover, to avoid injury, to improve, even to exercise properly.

Adults need seven to eight hours a night. As you get older, your need for sleep is not reduced, as many believe; rather, your sleep is more disturbed. As people age, they have greater trouble falling asleep and staying asleep, and they have a tendency to nod out unintentionally at odd moments. This is due to a change in their circadian rhythm: They get sleepier earlier in the evening but also awaken earlier the next morning. They may try to battle this by staying awake later into the night, only to find that they still wake up early, causing themselves yet more sleep deprivation.

Statistics show that in the twenty-first century just about everyone is sleeping less. Many factors are laying siege to the castle of your sleep, from work and family obligations to 24/7 entertainment options. But most of the shortfall happens because people let it, because sleep is a low priority, because deep down people think sleep is optional: "I can sleep when I'm dead." The truth is, they might get there a little faster, or a little more uncomfortably, if they don't get more shut-eye. (Be aware, though, that people who sleep *too much*—more than eight and a half or nine hours per night—have a higher rate of health problems and a higher mortality. This remains true even when other health-related parameters such as cholesterol level and blood pressure are taken into account.)

Most people believe they're fine on less sleep, but studies show that among pilots and truck drivers, missed sleep produces psychomotor impairment equivalent to the effect of a blood alcohol level above the legal limit. They also suffer from reduced memory and cognitive function and poor reflexes. Some people perform better than others when sleep deprived; scientists believe this may be a genetic gift. However, everyone displays some degree of reduced function when they're snoozing less.

And the effect is cumulative. According to research, missing an hour of sleep a night for a week affects your workout as dramatically as pulling an all-nighter. The first thing that goes is your mood, then your memory and ability to concentrate, then your reaction time. As the week drags on and you continue to miss that hour of sleep each night, your coordination during exercise diminishes, your performance level drops, and your reactions lag. Not a recipe for success, in exercise or in the rest of your life.

While You Sleep

While you sleep you are not simply giving your muscles and brain time off for good behavior. Your body during sleep is like a bustling after-hours warehouse store, forklifts whirring around with laden pallets resupplying empty racks with goods, workers sweeping up debris, and others laboring away on much-needed repairs. Fran Mason, M.D., coauthor of *The Force: The Proven Way to Fight Cancer Through Physical Activity and Exercise* and a physician who counsels elite athletes, has looked closely at the biology behind sleep. She notes that neuroscientists, doctors, and psychologists who study the biology of sleep have learned that there are a vast number of hormonal changes and neurochemical reactions that occur *only* while you sleep, and many of these have serious implications for your weight, your health, and your level of fitness. This is why you can't make up for missed sleep by drinking more coffee or popping vitamins. With so many systems under construction when you exercise, it's perhaps no surprise that adequate sleep becomes even more important.

A number of physiologic functions pivotal to good health, a trim waistline, and fitness are short-sheeted when you don't get enough sleep. "Research shows that you have fewer white blood cells in circulation when you slumber less. These 'natural killer cells' fight infection and represent the front line in your ability to ward off illness. They function best when you make your numbers regarding sleep. Also, research reveals that antibodies in the bloodstream produced in response to the flu vaccine are lower after six nights of partial sleep deprivation," says Dr. Mason. "Meanwhile, markers of inflammation go *up* as you sleep less. In general, inflammation is a bad thing for your health. It can result in a variety of problems for athletes, including pain, muscle soreness, arthritis, tendinitis, and other muscle and skeletal problems. Internally, inflammation is linked to conditions such as asthma, heart disease, and a number of other health problems."

Proper Sleep, Proper Weight

Scientists have found several reasons why sleep deprivation and obesity are also often bedfellows. According to Dr. Mason, two weight-regulating hormones are greatly controlled by the amount you sleep.

"The first is ghrelin, a small molecule manufactured by your stomach that rises between meals and falls rapidly right after you eat. Ghrelin levels elevate slowly as you sleep; when you don't sleep, ghrelin levels rise more sharply, by as much as 15 to 28 percent," says Mason. Research has linked this increase to a bigger appetite and weight gain. Studies have found that a lack of sleep can mean an additional five to fifteen pounds on the bathroom scale.

The second weight-regulating hormone tied to sleep is leptin, which is produced by your fat cells. "It helps you regulate hunger and the sensation of having eaten well by sending messages to your hypothalamus in your brain. Leptin levels also indicate your total body fat stores. The higher your levels of leptin, the higher your energy stores are perceived to be by your hypothalamus, and the lower your hunger and appetite will be," says Dr. Mason. "Leptin levels increase when you're eating excess calories. Leptin levels also rise *when you sleep*. When you cut back on sleep, your leptin levels drop almost 20 percent. This creates the same feelings of hunger you would have if you went on a diet that reduced your caloric intake by *30 percent*—essentially, mirroring the appetite you'd suffer by cutting your food intake by nearly a third or skipping one meal a day. In fact, studies show that hunger ratings are elevated when you are sleep deficient; so do your cravings for calorie-dense foods with high fat and carbohydrate content. That helps explain those late-night snacks."

Dr. Mason goes on to say that sleeping less also alters your thyroid metabolism by decreasing your pituitary gland's production of thyrotropin, a thyroid-stimulating hormone. "This may be linked to subtle changes in your resting metabolic rate during the day. If you cut your sleep back to four hours a night, you also experience a spike in the stress hormone cortisol and in your insulin resistance with glucose intolerance, the precursor to metabolic syndrome and diabetes," she says.

Human growth hormone (also known as somatotropin) is another bioactive molecule that is altered when you miss sleep. Like thyrotropin, it's produced by your pituitary gland. The greatest levels are produced at night, usually during early deep sleep in well-nourished, lean adults. Human growth hormone, which helps you maintain muscle mass by promoting protein synthesis and metabolizing fat, also promotes electrolyte and fluid balance.

In adults, hormone deficiency causes abdominal obesity, muscle weakness, and a change in body composition: In other words, you end up with less lean body mass and more fat. Levels of human growth hormone decrease naturally as you get older, but Dr. Mason points out that you can lessen its decline and help improve your body composition, muscle mass, and strength simply by *getting enough sleep*. Proper exercise causes the secretion of more growth hormone, which increases your bone metabolism and metabolism in general, thus bolstering your lean body mass even more.

Know the Techniques for Getting Enough Sleep

As you exercise more frequently, pay attention to your new and changing sleep requirements, then meet them. Maintain a regular bedtime to set and reinforce your circadian rhythm, your natural sleep cycle. You should also have a wake-up time that doesn't require an alarm clock; this helps guarantee that you're getting enough sleep. Working out (if it's not too late in the day) also makes you sleep better at night.

We Can Bank Sleep

Sleep, it turns out, can be banked like money. New research has revealed that, just as the loss of sleep is cumulative, so is getting an extra forty winks. If you cannot get sufficient overnight sleep, studies show that napping can be an effective way to make up the deficit. And extra sleep pays dividends if you take a nap *prior* to sleep loss. Got a late night planned? Take a nap earlier that day. Research shows that naps as short as ten to fifteen minutes and as long as two hours offer biological benefits; forty-five minutes seems to be about right when you are exercising.

Tapering

Tapering is another form of rest. Tapering is decreasing the exercise you do after a block of escalating amounts. Athletes employ this kind of rest prior to an event to stack the improvement-to-fatigue ratio in the favor of improvement. By strategically reducing your exercise leading up to a race, say, or a hiking trip, you maintain the improvements you've made to date, but don't push your body to new improvements and cause fatigue. This allows your systems to gather steam. Tapering is the gradual banking of energy, like the slow, deep breath you take in before you blow out the candles on a cake, or the one or two steps backward you take before exploding into a running leap. The most effective kind of tapering occurs when you reduce the amount of exercise you are doing by cutting back on the *volume* but not on the *intensity*. For example, if you normally power walk at high intensity for an hour a day, then three or four days before a major hike you would trim back your power walk to forty-five minutes but still do it at high intensity. The next day you would go for a half hour, the day after that for fifteen minutes, also at high intensity. Then you would take a rest day or two before the big hike.

By allowing your body to "rest" by tapering the volume of your exercise, you lower your fatigue overall. By exercising at the same intensity, however, you make sure you are keeping your systems firing on all cylinders as your big day approaches. This way, you will not lose your hard-won adaptations to high-intensity exercise.

Ideally, you should taper your exercise volume three days to one week before your event. If you are doing endurance sports (long hikes or bike rides, marathons or triathlons), your tapering should start about a week in advance; if you are preparing for an event in team sports, you should start two to three days before your event. To peak at the right time requires some tinkering, and the smaller your target, the more fine tuning you'll need, especially if there is a specific *day* on which you want to peak.

Days to Taper

How long you should taper within the advised range is determined by how quickly you respond to exercise and how quickly you recover. You can also get a sense of how quickly you detrain based on how quickly you improve. Do you require a good deal of time to get in shape? Or do you go out three times a week for three weeks and see improvement? If you respond quickly, you have a low threshold of trainability. (Eric does—he can go out five times and he becomes very strong.) If you have to work hard for your body to improve, then you have a high threshold. Most people adapt to exercise volume slowly, and lose those adaptations slowly. This is why it's important to do a certain volume of exercise every week; it establishes a firm base that's hard to shake. When it comes to intensity, most people adapt quickly but also lose the adaptations quickly. In general, the slower you build to a certain level of fitness, the longer it will stay with you. That's why, ideally, you want to build gradually and consolidate your fitness step-by-step.

Once you have an idea of whether you are quick or slow to train (and detrain), you can then experiment with blocks of tapering time during your exercise program. If you are a beginner, start by playing with different periods of tapering, then fine-tune depending on what your body tells you. Do you feel best after four days of tapering, for instance, or after twelve days of tapering?

We have professional athletes who want to do their last heavy workout three days before a race, or even two days or one day before. They say that if they don't work hard up to nearly the last minute, they feel sluggish. They feel as if there is no muscle "tension," and they start the race with the sensation that they are too relaxed. They like to start the race feeling that their legs have been working, or even with a little soreness, so they feel ready to fight. They don't like it when they feel too supple or too good at the start.

Other athletes are the opposite. They want to feel completely good and pain-free the day of the race, and they want their legs to feel supple and soft. They say, "I feel a little sluggish, but I know that midway through I will start to feel good." These athletes don't want to do *any* heavy workouts for five or six days before a race.

Studies show that after ten to twenty days without exercise most people will start to have symptoms of detraining on all physical fronts. In other words, you can't take three weeks off every month or you will always be starting from zero. We generally offer athletes a range for tapering within which to experiment to see what's ideal for them, because everyone recovers at a different pace. You need to discover ahead of time what works best for you personally. If you taper for a week and then have a great day, you are seeing the benefits of the right amount of rest via tapering. If you do so and do *not* have a great day, you have probably tapered too little; you need to adjust your tapering schedule next time. Experiment with varying periods of recovery with which you feel best and your body performs best, and individualize how you taper for your big event with reference to that.

Overtraining 101

Overtraining occurs when you don't give your body sufficient rest to allow recovery during an exercise program. Some of the symptoms of overtraining include:

- A general lack of energy throughout the day
- Underperformance, no improvement in your abilities, or a decrease in your abilities
- Low or no energy at the beginning of your workout

- Restless sleep or the inability to sleep
- Loss of appetite or an unusual desire to eat sugary foods
- Depression or anxiety

True overtraining is serious and needs to be addressed right away. Elite athletes have been known to lose entire seasons by not responding to overtraining soon enough. However, overtraining is not a pat diagnosis for everyone experiencing these symptoms. These same symptoms can also be rooted in simpler medical problems that are placing additional demands on your body.

When these symptoms occur, people who have learned that exercise brings improved performance, sleep, energy, vitality, and so on, often logically think that more exercise will relieve their symptoms. But redoubling their efforts only taxes their body further and makes their symptoms worse. In some people, this can spiral into a situation from which it is difficult to pull out.

On the other hand, resting—the answer for true overtraining—is not a cure for other maladies that may be causing the unusual fatigue and other symptoms. For these reasons, each case requires careful scrutiny. Here are some guidelines in assessing any symptoms of overtraining you might experience and some advice for how to work with your doctor in investigating other possible causes.

If you experience unusual exhaustion, fatigue, and underperformance, allergies should be your first suspect. You can have allergies with no obvious symptoms. What you will notice is that you simply don't perform well during certain times of the year. That does not mean that you should not exercise. Quite a few top athletes are well managed for their seasonal allergies, yet they still have months or seasons when their bodies simply don't perform well. So they skip the Tour of Italy, say, because it matches their allergy season. Michele Bartoli, a very strong one-day racer, and two-time World Cup winner, altered his season to be at his best outside of May and June even in years when he was doing very well. May and June were allergy season for him, and he didn't push himself when his body was vulnerable. In July and August, however, he would be allergy-free and peaking in time to win the World Cup races.

If you suspect you have seasonal allergies, see a doctor for a diagnosis and for help managing your symptoms. Like many top athletes, you may have to identify times of the year when you perform well, and design your exercise plan and goals accordingly.

Next, you will want to weigh whether your body composition could be contributing to your symptoms of fatigue and underperformance. People who are very muscular don't perform as well when it's hot and humid outdoors; ditto for people who carry extra fat. The additional effort required to keep cool can be taxing and cause unusual fatigue. These people do well in the cooler temperatures of spring or fall, or in an air-conditioned building. When the ambient temperature is cooler, they have extra protection from the cold, so they don't waste energy keeping warm. However, lighter people with no fat might feel fatigued and underperform as the days grow cool and their systems take on the additional burden of keeping warm as well as exercising.

A big factor that leads to the symptoms of overtraining is monotony. I'm Italian and I couldn't eat lasagna every day.

—Max

Monotony or lack of novelty in your exercise program is the next possibility to examine. We have talked about the important role your mind plays in performance. If your mind has checked out due to boredom with your exercise activities, this places an unusual burden on your body. Think of how much more grueling and tiring you find a task you have no interest in versus the ease with which you can do even very difficult tasks you are excited about. In an exercise program, this phenomenon can lead to the very same symptoms you would experience if you were overtraining.

A monotonous ongoing exercise routine also impacts your body on a physical level. If you do the same workout or try to maintain a very high level of fitness in one specialized arena year-round, your body is never allowed to rest or peak. This happens when athletes try to maintain the same level of fitness year-round. A cyclist, for example, might go straight from competing in road races in summer, say, to competing in cyclo-cross in the winter. She never allows herself a season to do something completely different, and she goes right into her next competitive season already bored and fatigued with no break in sight. It can also happen if you keep doing the same routine at the same intensity until you are nauseated by the very sight of your training shoes. If this is the case, take time off from that activity and choose a new one you're excited about.

The next possibility we consider as physicians is a subclinical viral infection. A very subtle infection can cause fatigue, muscle aches, and an overall feeling that your body is not a hundred percent, but it might impart no overt symptoms such as fever or chills. For this reason, you might think the symptoms are, again, a sign you need to exercise *harder*. Or you might think, A couple of workouts and maybe I can shake this, and you inadvertently make your infection last longer by training through it. If you think a subclinical viral infection might be the problem, you may not require any medication but simply a healthy diet and good hydration. You also need to moderate your exercise to maintain some of the intensity you are accustomed to, but to tax your body only twice a week to allow yourself rest until you have beaten your infection.

If you have worked with your physician and categorically eliminated all of these other possibilities, chances are that your fatigue and underperformance are indeed due to genuine overtraining. You will need to get a full assessment from a doctor, including a full physical evaluation and a psychological profile (this to measure your level of mental burnout). We do a physiologic profile to determine a person's muscle mass and blood parameters (this is where anemia or an iron deficiency without anemia may show up), we measure the level of blood lactate the athlete can build up, and at times we observe how some of his hormones respond to a stress test. If the athlete has a heart rate monitor, we download his information to look at his peak heart rate during exercise. If it isn't coming close to his usual maximum heart rate, this is a classic symptom of overreaching or overtraining. We probe for other information, too: How long does he sleep, and how well? What kinds of food does he crave? Does he feel anything new or different when he exercises? Answers to all of these questions can help us identify a case of overtraining.

I saw overtraining many times with elite athletes when serving as a team physician in races such as the Tour de France. Every morning I would go to each rider's room, knock on the door, and go in and take his blood pressure. If it appeared that the rider had been in the same position all night, I was assured he was fine. But if his blankets were twisted and thrown aside, or he had put the mattress on the floor, or he complained to me that the bed was too soft or the room too hot—if every little thing was bothering him—then I would wonder whether he had overtrained.

At mealtime, I would look for riders with insatiable appetites, especially those who were consuming cookies or other foods with sugar. I would also note riders who would leave a worrying amount of food on their plates, which is really unusual for a cyclist racing at that level of competition. Both of these ends of the appetite spectrum are classic symptoms of overtraining.

Still other athletes might come to me and report odd sensations: "I feel as if my legs are not pushing the same gear" or "I feel my body is different."

If I saw any of these things, I knew that in one or two days the cyclist wouldn't be able to finish the stage.

—Max

For elite athletes as well as the rest of us, the solution to real overtraining is not to give up completely but to manipulate your exercise program, particularly the amount of aerobic exercise you are doing each week. You do not want to quit completely and forfeit all of your hard-earned adaptations. Instead, you should *reduce the volume* of exercise you're doing while *maintaining the intensity* of your training. Making these adjustments will keep all of your improvements in a holding pattern while allowing your body to rest and recover.

If you have been challenging yourself with hard exercise or difficult races and events, you'll want to modify that and take break for a while. You might go back one step and rebuild more slowly, with more gradual increases than you attempted before.

That said, no overtraining problem is without complex considerations. What lies at the root of your possible overtraining is very individual and differs subtly from one person to another. As human beings, we are made out of the same material, but we need to be assessed as individuals. Once you have acknowledged a problem, you need someone to go to. If you suspect it's a medical problem, that person can be your regular doctor, a sports doctor, or an advice nurse; if it's an exercise problem it could be a good coach or trainer or a sports physical therapist. It's wise to establish a relationship with someone in advance, so he or she knows your history and your baseline, and so you're already part of the client base and will be a known entity if an issue arises.

It's important to recruit a trusted personal physician who deals frequently with athletes to be your partner in your quest for fitness. If you are overtraining, a doctor who is *not* accustomed to dealing with athletes might hear you complain of a loss of power, for example, and understandably tell you it's due to a lack of training or that you need to redouble your exercise efforts. Obviously, a misdiagnosis of overtraining like that can have serious consequences, but it happens all the time. Likewise, if you tell a physician that you feel pain doing a beloved activity, he may say, "Well, just stop doing it."

> It is vital for a physician to understand the characteristics of the athlete and the nuances of the sport when giving advice. I have found to develop this knowledge means spending time with the individual athletes and coaches and covering the competitions as a physician.
>
> —Eric

Once you reach out to a medical professional, make sure you are able to communicate with him. How well you can articulate your problem, pinpoint when it started, and rate its severity will come down to how much practice you've had in monitoring your own body, via your exercise diary among other strategies. (More on this in Chapter 10, "Better Motivation.")

You also want to look seriously at how you can reduce other stressors that might be contributing to the sum total of stress in your life. Exercise, as you know, in order to work, needs to stress your body. While you are stressing your body this way, you cannot afford to stress it other ways, or you are just piling it on. If you add too much work stress, commute stress, dieting stress, sleep stress, and family stress to exercise stress, you will find you get more colds, or muscle tears, joint pain, arthritis, even osteoporosis. While you exercise you owe it to your body to give it good, nutritious fuel; enough sleep; and adequate time to adjust to exercise stressors. To do so, it's often helpful to map your minimum and maximum workouts on a calendar in advance. Writing it down helps you internalize and commit to those numbers. You will be more honest with yourself, and less likely to go overboard, if you've already committed to what you will strive to achieve.

A good program helps keep you honest about increasing your exercise, yes, but it also helps moderate those increases so that you don't increase too quickly. That's why you must always heed the minimum and maximum exercise a program calls for, just as you would heed the maximum dosage on a prescription medication.

"I took care of my wheel as one would look after a Rolls-Royce. Often [my bike mechanic] would do the job for me without pay because, as he put it, he never saw a man so in love with his bike as I was."

—HENRY MILLER

8

better motion and gear

When you exercise, you are transferring power from your muscles to the pavement, the exercise machine, the paddle, the racket, the pedal. To apply the power of your engine as efficiently as possible (and to avoid mistakes that may cause injuries), you'll need to know a few things about biomechanics, an area in which Eric specializes. You'll also need to know how to troubleshoot classic activity-oriented injuries, if they should happen. Some basic guidelines on selecting the equipment you'll need on your road to fitness will come in handy, as will some tips about optimizing its use. Chief among that equipment is shoes.

SHOES

We have already discussed the way exercise exaggerates the burden carried by your lungs, your heart, and your muscles. Most types of exercise further multiply the impact on your feet. Who hasn't suffered the consequences of ill-suited shoes only after the shoes are "activity tested," say, on a day that required plenty of walking? Or in high humidity and heat? Or when carrying weight like a child or a backpack? When you walk or run, the forces (called joint reactive forces) at your knees are two to six times your body weight plus whatever weight you're carrying. So if you weigh 150 pounds and your backpack (or grandchild) weighs 50, that's 600 to

1,200 pounds at your knees with every footfall. Imagine the impact on your feet.

The level of support your feet have under conditions like these can make a big difference in how well, how often, and how happily you exercise. Beyond blisters, corns, and other superficial but debilitating foot injuries, a poor shoe choice can cause back pain, knee pain, and fatigue and have long-term effects on your knees, back, and hips. To be comfortable, safe, successful, and happy in your exercise program, good, carefully chosen shoes are crucial.

Shoe-in

Street shoes are divided into simple sizes, which may give you the impression that human feet vary only in length. In reality, however, feet come in myriad shapes and sizes, not as individual as a fingerprint or an iris, but nearly. To select a pair of shoes that will support you through the increased rigors of exercise, you need to be aware that your feet are a unique combination of:

- Gait
- Shape
- Width (heel and toe bed)
- Movement
- Volume
- Size

To choose the right shoe for exercise you likewise need to consider:

- The activity you plan to do
- Whether you will use your shoes indoors or out
- Whether you'll be using them in weather that is hot or cold, wet or dry
- Your body's circulation

Gait

Your gait is your manner of walking and involves variations in your hip, knee, and ankle flexion; coordination; and width between your knees.

Companies now make shoes that address almost every possible gait. The staff at specialty sports shoe stores are often trained in exercise kinesiology. They are there to help you determine the best shoe for your particular feet, and they can give you a gross evaluation of your gait.

First, Your Last

You will first narrow the array of available shoes to models whose shape fits the anatomy of your foot. Shoes are made using a solid form, called a last, around which the shoe is molded. A shoe's last can be compared to the fit of a suit (wide shoulders, narrow chest), and shoe companies tend to specialize in a particular shoe last. One company might make shoes designed for people who need wide toe boxes, or for people who have narrow heels, or for those whose feet are low or high in volume (thickness). Work with a salesperson at your athletic shoe store to find which companies use the proper last for you.

Shape

Most feet are one of three shapes. To find out your particular foot shape, wet your feet, then stand on a piece of paper. Now step off and look at the footprints.

- **Normal feet:** Your heel and forefoot are connected by a wide band that narrows slightly in between, where your foot arches. **Ideal shoes for you:** Those that feature cushioning and stability, with moderate control.
- **Feet with high arches:** Your heel and forefoot are connected by a very thin bridge. Feet with high arches don't absorb shock well and tend to supinate or under-pronate (they turn outward or don't turn inward). **Ideal shoes for you:** Those that are flexible and cushioning.
- **Flat feet:** Your entire foot leaves an imprint. Because you have a low arch, your foot rolls inward too much or pronates, which can lead to knee and hip misalignments. **Ideal shoes for you:** Those with motion control.

Motion: Shades of Gray

The best choice of shoe for you should now be narrowed further to the functional aspects of each shoe. These features control the motion of your foot. You can see the differences if you look at the shoes yourself: See the layers of cushion on the outside of a running shoe's sole? The white material is softer, the gray harder. If you pronate, you'll want a shoe with lots of gray on the inside (the arch). If you supinate (your foot rolls out), look for shoes with lots of gray on the outside.

Swell Solution

People with poor circulation tend to suffer swelling in their feet. The centrifugal force of pedaling or the impact forces of hiking, running, and walking push blood into the foot. With poor circulation, the blood is not returned efficiently to the heart, especially in activities where the calf muscles don't work very hard, such as cycling.

If you have noticed that after an hour of activity your shoes are too tight, we advise that you get fitted for shoes while wearing two pairs of socks. When exercising you can wear two pairs of socks for the first hour, then remove the second pair once your feet begin to swell.

Also, keep your toenails short and always cut them straight across to avoid ingrown nails, which tend to occur when your feet swell.

Weather Outlook

If you plan on wearing your shoes strictly indoors or in summer, choose those with a well-ventilated nylon upper. If your shoes are primarily intended for use outside or in wet and cold weather, choose a sturdy, less permeable upper made of vinyl or leather. If you will be running in water, you may want shoes with a Gore-Tex upper, but keep in mind that while these shoes will keep your feet dry, they will also make them hotter, which can cause blisters.

Activity Factors

The above shoe selection guide is perfect for the runner. For other activities, you will want to look for additional characteristics that make shoes better suited to your purposes.

Walking

Everyone should have a pair of shoes designed for walking. But to help avoid repetitive stress injuries, specialized walking shoes are especially *critical* for people who plan to make walking a routine. Do not make the mistake of using running shoes for walking; walking places unique demands on your foot. Walking shoes' soles are not as thick as those of running shoes because the impact on the foot is not as great, so less cushioning is required. Very often, walking shoe uppers are more substantial than those of running shoes. This makes them more resistant to rotational or longitudinal stresses that come about from walking on uneven surfaces and from frequent pivots and turns. As with running shoes, it's important that you replace your walking shoes every couple of months because the cushion in the soles wear out quickly.

Lifting weights

For lifting weights you need a shoe that provides good support and stability. The last thing you want is a narrow shoe with too much cushion in the heel. These features make it hard to maintain balance.

Aerobic dance, step aerobics, jumping rope, plyometrics

For very high-impact activities such as these, look for shoes that have some shock-absorbing qualities, and be sure to get new shoes every couple of months because under such duress, your shoes will lose the ability to absorb shock particularly fast.

Cycling

Even though your feet don't bear your full weight when cycling, the right shoe is as crucial in this sport as it is for other sports, if not more so, because in cycling all of the force is concentrated on one small area: your forefoot.

Determine your foot shape (as instructed above) and, with the help of staff at a bike shop, find a cycling shoe company that uses a last that accommodates your foot shape. Cycling shoe companies tend to specialize in one shoe last and do not often change, so once you find a company that works for you, stick with it.

People who get a burning sensation in the ball of their foot—a symptom of a condition that can be caused by the extreme pressure that cycling puts on the foot (and is eight to ten times more likely to occur in women than in men)—may require orthotics. If you do require orthotics, we recommend selecting cycling shoes that are wide enough to accommodate them. We further recommend a metatarsal pad (available at drugstores) to spread your toes. Recently a couple of cycling shoe companies have started to incorporate room for orthotics into their shoe designs. Be sure you don't get a shoe with a toe box that is too wide, however, or your foot will "float" within the shoe, which could lead to blisters.

Spinning

When doing a Spin class, the full load, again, is transmitted through your feet, so even though you are not *on* your feet, shoes are as critical as ever. In the beginning, it's not a bad idea to use cross-training shoes. They will offer adequate support. But if Spinning becomes a routine for you, get a nice pair of cycling shoes. Look for a pair with stiff soles; you shouldn't feel the pedal pushing through the shoe. (Also see the section on shoes for cycling.) If you are doing Spinning where you will need to walk across a concrete, vinyl, or wood floor, get mountain biking shoes with rubberized soles to avoid slipping.

Elliptical, treadmill, and general gym use

Cross-training shoes are the best choice for these uses. They have adequate cushion and good stability. You can use a treadmill for twenty minutes wearing these shoes and still have enough stability for weight training. Other shoes may be too soft to support your foot during weight training or not provide enough cushion for the treadmill.

Many Happy Returns

Because shoes are so individual, be sure you purchase your shoes at a place with a return policy that allows you to wear the shoes you select around the house for a while to truly test their fit.

And Repeat

After you have done all of your detective work and have found that one shoe that works best for you, note the name of the company and the model number so that you can purchase the same shoe in the future. The average life span of a pair of shoes is three or four months, or three hundred to five hundred miles. Do not buy further ahead than two years since the rubber has a limited life span and, even on the shelf, will break down with time.

Socks

If you are prone to blisters, choose socks that fit the contour of your foot rather than shapeless tube socks. A single wrinkle can cause a blister. If your feet get hot and sweaty with exercise, a thin sock with a thicker sock over it may alleviate rubbing and also help keep your feet dry.

> During my career, my Achilles' heel was my feet. I lived with blisters. Skates are extremely tight and a little fold in a sock could cause a blister that I couldn't get rid of for months. It was important that I find the correct shoes, and be ready with tape or moleskin whenever I felt a blister starting. I learned: Be aggressive with treating blisters before they start.
>
> —Eric

EXERCISE EQUIPMENT

Because exercise by its nature exaggerates movement, it also magnifies any problems or misfits you might encounter with the design of the equipment you are using. The following are a few of the more basic pieces of exercise gear and what to look for in them to avoid injury.

Racquets

To avoid injury in tennis and racquetball, the following three variables must be carefully chosen to fit your body and your game:

- The weight of the racquet (in tennis, for example, this can vary from 9 ounces to 12.5 ounces unstrung)
- Stringing tension (55 to 78 pounds per square inch)
- Grip size (in tennis, again, grip sizes range from 3⅞ to 4⅝)

If your needs do not match your racquet, you could develop wrist, elbow, or shoulder tendonitis as a consequence. Talk with a coach or trainer to get advice on purchasing a racquet appropriate for your level of play.

Weights

Having a weight set you can use at home makes muscle-strengthening exercise such as weight lifting less of a chore. You need not be intimidated; there are a number of compact weights on the market that are quite user-friendly.

If you invest in one weight set, especially dumbbells, beware of buying a set that requires you to physically add weight to a barbell (or remove it) as you do your different lifts. Why? Because it's human nature to become lazy and not change them. As a result, if you have forty-five pounds set to go, you may end up lifting forty-five pounds for everything—military presses, curls, flies, and abductions. There is great variation in the amount of weight you should be using for each type of lift. To make changing weight easy, get a rack of dumbbells ranging in weight from one to sixty-five pounds in five-pound increments. Nautilus also makes weight sets that allow you to dial in the weight you want; these have the added advantage of taking up less space as well.

Home Gym Equipment

Ninety to 95 percent of home gym equipment gathers dust in the guest bedroom. To avoid your piece of equipment suffering the same fate, the following guidelines might help.

- With gym equipment, you truly get what you pay for. Good quality will last you. If you can't afford new, look for a high-quality used piece.
- Before you buy, rent the item you are considering, or try it at a gym to be sure you will spend time on it.
- In advance, ensure that the store has a return policy that allows you to exchange the piece for something else if it doesn't work for you.
- Be aware that some Universal-type gym devices (those that feature a number of different functions on one piece) suffer from inconsistent resistance. With the ones that use pulley systems with spring or elastic bands, the resistance can be heavy at the start of the lift while momentum makes it light at the end. With spring-loaded systems, resistance can be light at the start and get heavier toward the finish. Try different products and find one that maintains consistent resistance throughout the range of the exercise.

Treadmills

Treadmills are a good tool for running or walking indoors. They are lower impact than running outdoors and offer good stride control. Your pace can be controlled on a treadmill, which can prevent you from opening your stride too much (important if you suffer from hamstring injuries), but still affords the hip extension and knee flexion of a good running workout. A treadmill is also convenient; it's no fun to be five miles out on a run, feel a twinge, and have to limp home.

In general, treadmills provide a good running bed for anyone who plans to run for an extended period of time, such as when you are training for a long event or a marathon. If impact is a big issue for you, anti-shock treadmills are available from several companies, including Precor, Nautilus, and TechnoGym.

Elliptical

These are hybrids, something between a stationary bicycle and a treadmill. Ideal for people who need to minimize joint forces.

Bicycle

Cycling is easy on your joints and a good tool for rehab from a knee, hip, or ankle injury. A good medium-priced bike is adequate for just about anyone, but it's important to spend time in picking up the right bike. Most bike shops are very good in providing the key information for a correct choice. You will want to go to a shop with a clear idea of the kind of riding you have in mind: long, hilly "solo" rides or fast and aggressive group rides? This will determine, together with your budget, the type and geometry of the frame and of the components used to build your bike. Your next step will be to focus on the frame size and the bike fitting. Most of us don't need a custom-made frame, but we all need a custom-made fit. The following are the key areas to concentrate on with regard to bike fit:

- The right saddle height and setback
- The correct crank arm length and a comfortable reach

This will make your experience more enjoyable and fun, which means you will ride more and longer.

Wind trainer

A wind trainer simply lifts the rear wheel of your bicycle, converting it into a stationary bike. It's possible to get a very good workout on a wind trainer. People have prepared for triathlons entirely on wind trainers, with little downside except perhaps lack of practice in bike-handling skills. For the sake of general fitness, wind trainers are ideal: You make the most of the time you have, and you eliminate outdoor hazards (cars, dogs, potholes, rain, snow, sun exposure, heat, humidity) and hassles (flat tires, no bathroom). Moreover, your bike stays very clean. And it is ideal for interval training. On a wind trainer you can gauge each interval exactly, while outdoors wind and changing terrain can conspire to vary each of your intervals.

CompuTrainer

If you want to get even more sophisticated with your indoor cycling, you can add a CompuTrainer to your fitness arsenal. A CompuTrainer is a computer-aided training device that offers you variable resistance as well as feedback on your speed, power, cadence, heart rate, and RPMs. It can even give you a "hill workout" by doing low RPMs in a big gear. You can also get software (to run on your computer while you ride your CompuTrainer) that lets you race your friends or the computer over courses that simulate the world championships, the Tour de France, or the Race Across America.

Portable Fitness Kit

Many fitness-seekers are hindered by the very real time constraints of work, family, and other obligations. It's wise to be prepared for those days when fitting in a run or an hour at the gym just isn't going to happen. To amplify your fitness, be ready to seize even small pieces of time—as little as ten minutes—by having at the ready a compact fitness kit. This is also handy for regular use in small spaces, such as an apartment, an office, or a hotel room. Indeed, in two square meters you can do a lot.

Jump rope

Jumping rope is an ideal way to get a concentrated aerobic workout with minimal equipment, space, and time. You can keep a jump rope tucked in a filing cabinet and use it during your breaks at work, packed in your suitcase for that last-minute business trip, or on a hook next to the back door to squeeze in some aerobic bursts while your kids play in the sandbox.

Look for a jump rope that has rotating handles and is not too lightweight. Be sure to get one designed for adults (children's jump ropes tend to be too short and too light). To assess the proper length, hold the handles and stand with the jump rope trapped under the arches of your feet. Your elbows should be bent at no more than a ninety-degree angle. If the jump rope is too long, shorten it by knotting the rope near the handles.

Avoid jumping rope if you have heart disease, Achilles tendon problems, plantar fasciitis, or any other condition that makes jumping an issue. For everyone else, it's a great way to include some aerobic exercise in an otherwise sedentary day.

Start by doing very short intervals, jumping rope for fifteen seconds, then resting for fifteen seconds. Work your way up to one minute of jumping rope with thirty-second rests, with the goal of eventually jumping rope for three minutes continuously.

For a quick overall workout, divide three-minute intervals of jumping rope with sets of push-ups and abdominal crunches.

Resistance stretch bands or surgical tubing

This is an underrated star in anyone's indoor workout kit. A resistance band is an ideal means of exercising muscles for several reasons. Its level of resistance increases with the degree of muscle contraction, and it adapts to the angle of the joint. In other words, as you pull it toward you, for example, the band gets harder to pull. This is the opposite of what happens with machine or free weights, where your maximum effort occurs at the beginning of the contraction, but as you pull the weight toward you, momentum takes over and it becomes easier. With elastic bands there is no momentum to bail you out; you must exert energy the entire time.

A number of companies now make stretch bands specifically for exercise. Some feature a bar for curls or an overhead military press; others can be attached to a door. Exercise stretch bands also vary in levels of resistance, from easy to super high. Don't make the mistake of buying a resistance band that's too hard for you to stretch. A good substitute for commercial resistance stretch bands is surgical tubing, which is sold by the foot at medical supply stores. This tubing also comes in a variety of resistances but without handles; however, you can easily knot them in loops. Or you can try Max's favorite, a used bike inner tube. (Mind the valve.)

When using bands, always be careful that they are firmly anchored so they won't come loose and cause you injury.

Rules for Walking

I like the convenience of working out at or near home, not having to travel somewhere. It's nice to have the opportunity to exercise right outside my door.

—Eric

Walking is a good general activity you can always keep in your back pocket, to do on days when life conspires to prevent you from doing any other aerobic activity. Pack your shoes to walk the stairs at work during lunch or when traveling. When you are in an unfamiliar place, ask tourist information, hotel staff, coworkers, or someone else with good local knowledge to point out streets, trails, or malls that are safe for a jaunt. At home, at work, or traveling, here are a few guidelines for keeping yourself safe:

- Avoid running or walking alone; stick to times of day when others will be around.
- Tell someone your route and when you expect to be back.
- During your run, don't be distracted by listening to music or talking on your cell phone. Instead, stay aware of your surroundings.
- Always carry an ID and $20 for a snack—or, notes Eric, cab fare back.

Selecting an Exercise Facility

If you are considering joining a health club or gym, here are a few general guidelines in assessing your candidates:

- Look for a place that is very convenient for you to use, either near your home or workplace or on the way to work.
- Make sure the place is clean (equipment, workout rooms, pool, showers, sauna).
- Check the credentials of the trainers on staff. Staff trainers should also have a good rapport with members.
- Talk with members and get their feedback regarding the club.
- Ask whether the gym limits the number of members. If it does not, you may end up waiting during peak hours to use equipment.

- Determine the days of the week and times of day you are most likely to use the gym (on your way to work, on your way home, during lunch hour, while the kids are in school). Then visit the gym at those times. How busy is it? Are the people there the kind of folks you'd feel comfortable working out beside? Some women feel more comfortable working out in a same-sex facility, for instance, and some serious bodybuilders prefer a gym that caters primarily to bodybuilders.
- If you plan on taking classes (such as an aerobic, step, or other impact class) or intend to play basketball or volleyball, look for a gym with a floor that's not concrete (or linoleum or wood on concrete). Concrete magnifies the shock of high-impact activities and can cause injuries consistent with long-distance running: stress fractures, tendonitis, patella-femoral syndrome, arthritic pain, and hip stress fractures. The floor should instead be made of any one of several materials that are slightly spongy to absorb loading properly. Ask to walk on the floor you'll be using for high-impact activity. Test the feel of the floor by jumping on it. The right floor should offer some resistance but absorb shock.

Selecting a Personal Trainer

A personal trainer may seem like a luxury, but hiring someone for even one or two sessions to guarantee that you are lifting properly or using gym equipment correctly can help you avoid a world of hurt. If a coach has achieved success with one athlete, ask yourself whether it's the coach who is very good—or the athlete. Many coaches are good scouts but are not good at nurturing talent. They know how to *select* people, but not how to *develop* them. Look for someone with a full range of people they have coached to success.

For a longer-term relationship, the choice is more personal, but the following is a general checklist designed to help you make your decision:

- Check to see whether the trainer is a member in good standing of a training association.
- Ask to talk to some of his clients, and get feedback from them.
- Personal trainers run the gamut from those who work with couch potatoes to those who train elite athletes. Ascertain that the trainer is appropriate for your level of fitness and can accommodate your schedule.
- Ask about his philosophy in motivating people. Some people want a

personal trainer who will be in their face, others want someone very supportive.

- Ask about the trainer's level of involvement. Some people want a trainer who will give them a program and leave them to their workout; others want their trainer there every day.
- Ask whether the trainer is comfortable with your sport, be it cycling, dance, lifting, or basketball.
- Ask about her long-term program, the amount of variety she can offer, and the ways she can keep you stimulated and motivated. For example, is she willing to run with you five days a week for five weeks and then get you into some kind of organized aerobic sport, such as basketball or soccer?

What's Your Sport?

We may look at a champion cross-country skier and think that the sport gave his body that long, lean look. But in fact it's often the reverse—it's people who have long, lean bodies that do well in cross-country skiing.

Throughout the sporting world, certain shapes seem to dominate. Indeed, various physiological factors affect how you transfer power in sports, so certain body types do better in each sport than others. You can look at the athletes who are successful in their sports and get a good general idea of what anthropometric features allow them to do well.

Experts (sports medicine doctors, orthopedic surgeons, family doctors) can help parents identify the sports for which their child is best suited via nothing more than an X-ray of the child's hand. Other anthropometric measurements also yield clues. In fact, you can get a sense of "your sport" simply by looking in the mirror. If you have:

- Long femurs: Try cycling, skating.
- Big feet and long arms: Try swimming.
- Stocky body, short arms: Try weight lifting. (You don't have to push the weight up as high as someone with long arms.)
- Short with stocky body: Try skiing. (Strong, thick, compact people have a lower center of gravity; the greater lever arm of taller people means more injuries.)
- Lean body: Try cross-country skiing.
- Hypermobility (great flexibility): Try swimming, gymnastics, yoga.

- ■ Stiff joints: Try running. People with stiff joints have less tendon elasticity, and so—like a tighter rubber band—spring back better. These folks can rely on their tendons to propel them rather than relying simply on sheer muscle power. (For this reason, some Kenyan runners don't even stretch before running in order to maintain strong elasticity in their tendons.)
- ■ Good upper-body strength or overall fitness: Try mountain biking.

Optimizing Motion

Repetition equals refinement. To improve your performance and reduce injuries, you will want to make your motion as efficient as possible. And practice does, in fact, make perfect.

When you bicycle, for example, muscles in your legs, abdomen, and chest contract and relax in a dance with one another that produces the movement that propels you forward. The choreographer of this dance is your brain. Improving the communication between choreographer and dancers proves to be very valuable. Having worked for years with cyclists of all levels, we know that maximum muscle strength has little to do with the ability to push hard and long on the pedals. Champion cyclists, for example, cannot leg-press as much weight as a weight lifter or a bodybuilder. Cyclists instead utilize efficiency in pedaling to maximize what muscle strength they have.

An experienced cyclist's brain has been programmed to contract and relax her muscles very precisely so they are never working against one another. Rehearsal in recruiting her muscles programs the brain over time. Think about a beginning skier: She exerts tremendous upper-body energy to compensate for the movement of her skis. Likewise, someone who's just started riding a bike is always in the wrong gear; he fatigues quickly, then tries another gear. Like a beginning driver, they both give it too much gas and then brake too hard. After years, however, you shift before the hill, and you stop pedaling before the turn so you don't have to brake. An automatic connection develops between your legs, hands, and eyes. Through multiple stimulations of the required movements over time, your brain learns to do it without conscious effort.

Your brain controls movement by sending a signal along a nerve to your muscle, causing your muscle to fire in the right sequence. Relax, contract, relax, contract. On and off, on and off. When bicycling, for example, if your brain is up to speed and firing with high efficiency, your quads (the muscles on the front of your thighs) contract to push down the pedal while your hamstrings (the muscles on the back of your thighs) relax.

Sounds simple, but this simultaneous contract-relax sequence is actually very complicated for your brain to pull off. If your brain has not had lots of practice, the muscles won't be synchronized. Your quads will contract and push down the pedal while your hamstrings are still contracted. This is like driving a car with the brakes on—definitely learner's-permit status. This internal resistance happens below your conscious level, but what does rise to the level of consciousness is a sense that you are wasting energy.

The solution lies in repetition, and the payoff is cumulative, adding up over the course of your lifetime. Those internal biomechanical resistances are reduced by every mile, stride, and lap you do, as you add to your lifetime totals of riding, walking, running, swimming, and so on. At a certain point, your body will top out on its ability to improve utilization of oxygen, but improvement will continue. How? Your body perfects your exercise *economy* via repetition, which allows you to perform the motion using less energy.

Your brain does this by optimizing resources, using increasingly more streamlined signals to and from your muscle. The muscle and the nerve that serves that muscle work as a team called a motor unit. As you practice an activity, you learn how to recruit or call on the right motor unit, depending on the muscular contraction you need. Each time you practice the activity, you recruit or call upon more muscle fibers to contract or relax; thus more motor units are involved and the right motor units are reinforced. This means more circuits and more connections, which smoothes the delivery of information. Ultimately, your movement becomes more precise. In lab efficiency tests, the most efficient cyclists, for example, are not the professionals who ride twenty-five thousand miles a year, but the cyclists over age sixty who have pedaled many more total miles over the course of their lives because they have the gift of repetition under their belt. And as their body has lost strength through age, they have unconsciously learned to compensate by pedaling more and more wisely and economically.

You might want to try workouts designed to gain biomechanical efficiency. If you are a cyclist, ride a fixed-gear bike. On this kind of bike, the pedals spin with the tires whether you're exerting energy or not; if you wanted to coast, you'd have to remove your feet from the spinning pedals. To improve your biomechanical efficiency, you keep your feet attached to the pedals so your feet move in circles with them. As this happens, your brain learns, *This is a circle*. (Pedaling a regular bike with one leg also improves your pedaling efficiency.)

If your pedaling is not efficient, it will be evident on a fixed-gear bike: With each rotation you will experience a tiny bump on the saddle. On the basis of this negative feedback, your brain will work harder to integrate the information it's getting from the pedals, in order to control the motion and avoid bumps or pains in your knees and your muscles.

To improve your efficiency in running, walking, or other sports, try performing the activity (running on a treadmill, for example) in front of a mirror. There are also sport-specific drills. The more difficult the technique required to do the sport, the more you can gain by improving your efficiency. Swimming provides a good example. If you throw someone who's never been swimming into the water, he will be *very* inefficient, very likely using every muscle in his body just to stay afloat. After a few swim lessons, however, he'll show a vast improvement in efficiency. He will be much better—smarter—at controlling his body and unconsciously concentrating his efforts on using only the muscles that will do the most good.

At the opposite end of the spectrum is walking, a sport that requires so little technique that toddlers can do it. As a result, you don't improve that much, even over a lifetime. Cycling straddles the spectrum midway between swimming and walking—it's not as complicated as the butterfly stroke, but it does require balance, the ability to ride in a straight line, and the coordination to push on the pedals. In general, know that better efficiency will happen on its own just by your performing your favorite activities repeatedly.

INJURIES

Exercise Discomfort

Practice doesn't just make perfect, it also makes more comfortable. Continuing to exercise will actually "immunize" you against the discomfort you feel when you first start out. The sensations you feel change as your body develops the capacity to handle the load. Experience at exercise transforms the early trials into a feel-good experience. But because of the fear of those initial sensations when trying new activities, most people veer off toward sports that they have always done and avoid areas of exercise they have never or rarely explored. Ironically, these unexplored areas often are their missing link to balanced, overall fitness and often hold the promise to the greatest leaps in benefit as well.

I was nervous before races, but not about winning or losing. I would get nervous about the fact that every time you race, you're racing against the clock, and you have to be able to dig deep. I got nervous about how much suffering [there would be]—how much it was going to hurt.

—Eric

Pushing yourself athletically may at times be uncomfortable, but the kind of displeasure you experience when you are in good shape differs substantially from the sensations you feel when you are out of shape. When first starting out, the discomfort of exercise can be, well, uncomfortable. The burning in your muscles and gasping for breath feel desperate because your systems can't deliver all that the exercise is demanding. However, as you grow fitter, all of your systems get better at delivering what you need. Your lungs, heart, and blood have ramped up; your brain and muscles have synchronized and become more efficient; your mitochondria have increased in size and number to dish out more energy; and your body has learned to better utilize that energy, better triage your blood flow, and better store glucose.

It seems like *every* time I start to exercise I think I'm too tired, it hurts too much, I'm not going to make it—even on days I end up having my best workouts. So when I start moaning to myself, "The water's too cold," or "The hill is too steep," or "I just don't feel like it," I remind myself that after the first ten minutes, I'm always comfortable and happy. And sure enough, ten minutes into it, I'm fine. So those initial fears of discomfort? They don't mean anything.

—DeAnne

At this point your systems will crave use. Your body will actually *want* to be challenged further. Exerting yourself simply becomes a matter of taking the effort up a notch. Striving for more will feel healthy, even exhilarating. In fact, top athletes often confess that during peak efforts they feel *pleasure*. And it makes sense—their body is running on all cylinders, it's doing what it's been primed to do. That explains in part why some people look forward to and truly enjoy exercise.

Managing Discomfort

That said, if you experience exercise discomfort, there are measures you can take to better manage it.

First, exercise pain is always a combination of the following factors:

- Your level of fitness
- The intensity of the exercise
- Your motivation to keep exercising
- The degree to which you *perceive* you are suffering
- The degree to which you can tolerate the exercise

The sensations of breathlessness and burning muscles, for example, correlate with the intensity of your effort. When you're out of shape, numerous receptors all over your body beg your brain to slow down. *I can't maintain this.* As you beef up each system, however, fewer receptors holler for mercy because your systems aren't working so close to their maximum capacity. As you keep at it, the sum of the signals screaming at your brain will level off considerably and the more pleasant sensations will be able to rise to a conscious level. And, if walking three miles an hour used to feel horrible, once you are walking five miles an hour regularly, three miles an hour won't register on your discomfort radar. You will suddenly understand why people exercise to unwind and feel tranquil. Not long after this you'll discover the real secret: how much fun exercise is.

Your brain also will become trained to manage fatigue. So even if 70 to 80 percent of your maximum is uncomfortable when you start out, once you've been doing it for a while, you will no longer perceive discomfort. Your brain will actually interpret the signals from your muscles and lungs differently. The signal that was once an emergency siren is now just a familiar signpost: *Oh, we've pushed this hard before. We know what to do; it'll be okay.*

Your level of motivation will also color how the signal is interpreted. Here's where the chatter going on in your cerebral cortex is cardinal to your fitness: It's responsible for telling you how long you *want* to push yourself. *I can hold this for another thirty seconds.* This may have been a factor in Lance Armstrong's victories; he's very good at motivating himself through higher levels of discomfort. That's what the best athletes in any sport have in common, and the one who pushes longer than the others is the one who will win. But what is important for you to know as you exercise is that the level of signals coming from your body has a value—a number from one to ten, say—but the message from your *cortex* can modify that value, given the motivation. A seven one day can feel like a ten if it's raining and you don't want to be out there. Other days it can feel like a three, if you're having a wonderful time with friends.

Some scientists now believe your body signals you to stop well before the point of exhaustion, to keep a little in reserve in case you need to run from that lion in your evolutionary past. But each time you can motivate yourself to push *through* that point, your body sets the limit a little higher. Thus, the signal that you once perceived as fatigue—*I can't go any farther*—is now perceived as *okay, but I know I can go a lot farther*. What was once your threshold is now an open door.

Evaluating what is going on with your body will be important to your program. It's much easier to view a change objectively when you have numbers. To do this you need a ruler—an "ouchometer"—for measuring your complaints. The following tips will give you a means of assessing your aches and pains objectively and help provide a way to articulate your body's responses and their severity to others when necessary.

In a notebook I keep track of how much weight I'm lifting and how I'm feeling:

- Bench-press—how much?
- How does it feel doing crunches?
- After how many reps do I first start to feel the burn?
- How long does it take me to recover and do another set?
- How do I feel after ten sets? After five?

—Eric

When embarking on a new exercise program, even if you're used to exercise, you will experience many new sensations. Keep a journal to increase your awareness of the signals your body gives you. Each time you exercise:

- Write down the date and time of your workout and its intensity.
- Record any unusual physical sensations.
- Gauge how you perceive the workout on a scale from one to five, with one being very easy and five being very strenuous.

■ Rate any muscle soreness or fatigue you feel subsequent to the workout, also on a scale from one to five, with one being nonexistent and five being severe.

■ When judging your performance during a workout you wedged into a particularly busy day, factor in the stresses of work, family, and other obligations. (If you worked late, you're not likely to have a lot of energy. If you've had a few nights of interrupted sleep, you aren't going to feel as invincible.)

■ List any other life stressors present that day: missed sleep, missed meals, extreme weather, long hours at work, worries, illnesses, and how severe the impact of those issues are, again rating them from one to five.

To keep track of how you feel during your exercise sessions, you can make copies of the following chart. (Photocopy this, or download blanks from our Web site: www.fasterbetterstronger.com.)

Daily Exercise Diary

Date and time of workout: _____   Intensity: _____

Rate the impact of each, 1 to 5, 1 being nonexistent and 5 being severe.

Any unusual physical sensations: _____

Rate above sensations: 1   2   3   4   5
    Nonexistent   Severe

Rate workout: 1   2   3   4   5
    Very easy   Very strenuous

Rate muscle soreness and fatigue:

           1   2   3   4   5
    Nonexistent   Severe

Other stressors:

  Missed sleep _____   Travel _____   Illness _____

  Extra work hours _____   Worries _____

  Extreme weather _____   Missed or poor meals _____

This type of exercise journal aids your success in an exercise program on several levels. First and foremost, it forces you to think carefully and consciously about these factors, which will make you more sensitive to them and how they impact your motivation, your exercise, your performance, and your health. Keeping a journal also creates a record of your exercise sensations over time, which is useful for comparison or for discerning patterns. You will notice when something that normally feels "2" suddenly feels "5," for example. Or a problem that has been nagging you for an inordinate amount of time may emerge—you may see that you've been noting "4"-level soreness in one joint for the past two weeks. The journal ratings also give you a concrete number with which to objectively assess your injuries or illnesses, and supply the words for articulating any potential problems and their severity to your doctor, should you need to. Doctors love 1 to 5.

I keep an exercise diary. It's worthwhile to monitor your feelings relative to the workout itself.

—Eric

Some people depend upon a coach so that he can adjust their training to account for other factors in their life. There's also lots of training software that can give you a general idea of what to do, and can lay out the necessary external load in a very graphic way using certain criteria. But a computer can never modulate the load on a daily basis, depending on your day. On a given day, the program may dictate an hour on the treadmill at moderate intensity. But maybe your heart rate is not going up; maybe you're fatigued or a little sore. Perhaps you missed a workout or two earlier in the week. What to do? Back off completely? Redouble your efforts? A computer cannot tell you.

But your diary can give you clues. Looking back through your scribbled daily entries, you will discern patterns: You're always fatigued at this point in the week. Or you failed to take your rest days and therefore have overdone it, which means all of your biologic systems need to rebuild and recover.

In addition to fatigue, you also need to ensure that your problems are not dietary, that you are providing your body with the right fuel for someone who is exercising. This means lots of wholesome carbohydrates, in addition to other nutrients. (See Chapter 5.) You may also want to rule out iron deficiency through a blood test. Iron deficiency is the most common micronutrient deficiency in the United States and in other developed countries. Globally, an estimated 1.25 billion people are affected. In young female athletes involved in endurance sports, the iron-deficiency rate is as high as 50 percent.

As you know, iron is necessary to make hemoglobin, the primary molecule in red blood cells responsible for the transport of oxygen. When it comes to low iron, your performance goes into the red zone before the iron deficiency is advanced enough to cause real "anemia" and symptoms can develop. If you have an iron deficiency lasting long enough to cause anemia, your red cells will appear smaller than normal. They will also be paler in color; this reflects their low hemoglobin content.

If you come in complaining of fatigue and your iron test results (in particular your ferritin level) fall within the very lowest range of normal recommended by the Centers for Disease Control, a doctor may say your blood test is normal. But for us, when working with people who are getting fit, the low range of normal is significant when it comes to iron, especially if you are a female endurance athlete, you are training hard, you have heavy menstrual cycles, you follow a vegetarian diet, or, most important, you are unusually fatigued. Worsening performance in an athlete is often explained by pure iron deficiency, even without anemia. So you need to ask your doctor for the specific results of the test—not simply whether you scored within the range of normal. Be aware that, if your doctor will start you on iron supplementation therapy, you will feel better before your blood count improves.

Getting to Know You . . .

On a deeper level, you must also learn to communicate what is going on in your body. Consider the following:

1. How aware are you of your physical sensations while you exercise?
2. How well do you recognize and describe your aches and pains, your injuries and fatigue?
3. How do you gauge the severity of your aches and pains? Do you brush them off unless they are life threatening? If not, how do you acknowledge the physical problems and treat them?

The importance of good communication to the success of an exercise plan perhaps doesn't have the same scientific research behind it that our other principles do, but we have learned through experience that it's vital. In fact, the communication component of exercise is too often overlooked. Some things you can measure in a lab or with self-administered tests every so often, but on a day-to-day basis you need to be able to monitor *yourself* by being aware of your body and its signals. And that requires good communication between your mind and your body, as well as with your coach if you have one.

You need a system for knowing when changes in your body require attention, and how to best articulate those changes to the right people in order to get the attention you need. You need to describe and rate those sensations. You also need a gauge.

Recognize a Problem and Rate the Problem

Anyone who has seen a cold circulate through a group of people knows that individuals can assess responses from their bodies in vastly different ways. Some are on their deathbed with the sniffles; others are out chopping wood or doing surgery. It is no different when it comes to asking people to rate their responses to exercise.

Likewise, some people are adept talkers—they are very good at describing how they are doing, how they feel, what they need; other people are much more reserved. In fitness there are people who never complain, and there are people who complain all the time.

> When I was a family doctor, I dealt with so many people, all with different personalities: people who were histrionic or dramatic, people who were very shy, people who were depressed. Each conveyed information differently. But it's important to note that they also "heard" information differently. Some people let everything roll right off. Others were less resilient; they didn't spring back easily from the dings of life. This was due in part to what they told themselves about the information they received.
>
> —Max

Which are you? Be honest. Understanding your basic temperament serves you well as you coach yourself in exercise. There is no better or worse way to be. In fact, it can be said that both extremes stem from a lack of sensitivity to the nuances of the body.

> I was reserved—very aware of the physical sensations while training, but reserved. I loved to train hard and would not give in to exhaustion. I liked the feeling of fatigue during training and felt satisfied that it was a good workout day when I was exhausted at night.
>
> —Eric

What seems sheer exhaustion, great hunger, or significant pain for one person wouldn't register on the radar of another person. But that doesn't mean the latter is a better, tougher athlete—she could easily push herself too far. Likewise, the person who interprets every response from his body as cause to call an ambulance, call his adviser, or call off training will suffer, too: He could skip exercise unnecessarily or complain so often that his doctor might be unable to recognize an injury that requires medical attention.

Whatever your personality, if you develop a localized chronic pain that is persistent with exercise, it might be wise to seek medical advice to rule out such problems as a stress fracture.

The bottom line is that you have to know when you have a problem, you have to be able to rate the problem, and you have to be able to communicate the problem to an adviser when necessary. But how to know when it's necessary? To determine this, you have to first know who you are: the knight in Monty Python ("It's just a flesh wound," he says of his arm being torn off)? Or Henny Penny ("The sky is falling," she cries when she gets hit on the head with a seed)? Or someone in between? In your role of self-coach, you have to know the temperament of the athlete with whom you are dealing, yourself, so you can readily distinguish between an injury and an owie.

AVOIDING INJURIES

There's nothing like an injury to hinder (or halt) your exercise progress. How you execute your activity may prevent injury. Here are some basic tips on avoiding the most common sports injuries.

All activities

Don't neglect stretching. Stretching does not impart the normal soreness people associate with exercise, so they don't believe stretching is accomplishing anything. Thus it's the first thing people delete from their exercise routine. However, stretching is central to avoiding injury. It increases blood flow to your tendons and muscles, which helps avoid strains. It also lubricates your joints. Even an activity with a small range of motion, such as cycling, requires stretching: If you fall, you won't pull muscles if you're limber.

> When I was skating, we had two or three workouts a day and we spent fifteen minutes stretching before and after every workout. That adds up to a lot of time stretching. But that's how necessary it is.
>
> —Eric

Weight lifting

Good lifting mechanics are essential. Have someone with experience show you proper lifting form. Keep your back nice and straight and the weight over your center of gravity as you go up and down. To avoid lower-back issues, do squats holding the weight lower and closer to your lumbar spine (lower back) rather than at shoulder level. The lower height of the weight lessens the risk of lumbar spine injuries.

To avoid abdominal strains, be cautious about overdoing it. Progress slowly with the amount of weight and number of repetitions. Remember, when you finish you should feel as if you could do more—but don't. You won't feel the effects of the muscle work until twenty-four to forty-eight hours later.

Couple your weight training with other abdominal and core exercise such as Pilates.

Using belts for lifting helps with mechanics by keeping your back rigid, but most people would benefit more from using them less. They are essentially a crutch that eventually weakens your core muscles, which are the muscles you need to strengthen to avoid back and abdominal strains.

Swimming, racquetball, handball, or tennis

Mechanics are important with activities requiring overhead motion, like swimming, golf, racquet sports, and even some weights. To avoid shoulder injuries in racquet sports, work on your overhead and ground strokes and your serve. Have a coach assess and advise you on your form.

If you experience shoulder pain, stay in the "safe zone" when you exercise: Keep your hands shoulder level and below. This avoids putting stress on your shoulders. When lifting, lie on your back on a bench, with your feet higher than your head, and do bench presses toward your feet. When swimming, do the breaststroke or crawl, or use a kickboard. And vary your stroke.

To guard against wrist and elbow injuries, concentrate on good technique; make sure you have a racquet with the right string tension, weight, and grip size. Be aware that the Western grip puts more stress on your wrist than do other grips.

Golf

Make sure you have the correct shaft stiffness, grip size, and clubhead weight. Proper technique is also necessary, so have a pro assess yours. Also, practicing on grass rather than a mat will be easier on your wrists and elbows.

Cycling

Make sure your bike fits your body correctly. There are standard bike fit parameters, but there are also small adjustments that can be made to address individual issues.

Running

Overuse injuries are the most common runners' complaints, and many of these can be avoided by staying away from hard running surfaces, varying the route you run, and getting shoes that fit your running style. **If you do develop localized pain that is persistent with exercise, it might be wise to seek medical advice to rule out such problems as a stress fracture.**

Muscle Soreness

Muscle soreness twenty-four to forty-eight hours after you exercise is a good sign; it means that you have challenged your muscles and are getting stronger. This is called delayed onset of muscle soreness (DOMS), and everyone experiences it, even elite athletes. Here's how to handle DOMS:

1. Heat (in the form of a hot shower or bath, sauna, hot tub, or hot pad) may relieve some of the soreness by bringing more blood to the site.
2. Avoid taking an antiinflammatory for DOMS. They have been shown to delay recovery.
3. Follow your regular exercise schedule. Skipping a session could prolong your recovery. Studies show that active recovery works best with DOMS.
4. Before your next exercise session, do a five-minute warm-up, such as running in place, then stretch thoroughly.

If muscle soreness prevents you from participating in your regularly scheduled workout, this is a sign that you have pushed yourself too far and need to bring your exercise routine down a notch—not quit completely, just ease off a little.

Troubleshooting aches and pains before they lead to chronic overuse injuries:

1. Try to identify the mechanism that has produced the soreness, and avoid it for two weeks. If you're doing a number of activities, keep a diary to track your workouts. If, for example, you do a Spin class every Tuesday and you always notice the soreness on Wednesday mornings, substitute the class with another activity for two weeks.
2. While resting, you can use an antiinflammatory medication (Motrin, ibuprofen, Aleve, Advil, and prescription Celebrex) acutely to treat the symptoms. *Do not use NSAIDS on a regular basis to mask symptoms and continue the activity.*
3. After taking two weeks off from that specific activity, try it again, without antiinflammatories. If soreness returns and persists and it's an activity you don't want to stop, seek expert advice from a doctor, coach, or athletic trainer.

4. Try modifying your technique, using different equipment, and doing strengthening exercises. The expert you consult should be able to offer guidance.

5. If after trying all of the above, the pain persists, you may need to turn to a different activity.

6. If you haven't spoken to someone and you're taking antiinflammatories on a regular basis, you definitely need to seek expert advice. There may be long-term consequences to continuing the activity that's injuring you, and taking antiinflammatories chronically can lead to other health issues. These include liver failure and stomach bleeding (which can be fatal yet show no warning signs). If necessary, cycle onto the drug for the weekend, then off again on Monday for the week.

7. You may want to try Tylenol (acetaminophen). Some people don't realize that Tylenol is good for joint pain and muscle pain, but it is as effective as antiinflammatories and probably safer for most individuals if taken as directed.

8. If exercise triggers arthritis pain, glucosamine is worth trying. There isn't clear scientific evidence, but anecdotal evidence suggests that it helps. To test its effectiveness for yourself, try it for two months (there are no known side effects), then stop for a few weeks and see if symptoms return.

Risk Factors

After you have done the risk factor assessment in Part Two, if you had one or more stars but have had no event or diagnosis, check with your doctor first and see if you may begin to exercise. If so, we urge the following:

If your one risk factor was cardiovascular *in nature (such as high blood pressure):*

■ Perform aerobic activity at mild to moderate intensity and increase the volume very, very slowly.

You are among the people who can benefit most from our program. This type of program has been shown to reduce high blood pressure and is in fact shown to be negative risk factor—you subtract it from other risk factors you might have.

If you experience shortness of breath, chest pressure, chest pain, light-headedness, or if you're a woman and experience shortness of breath or the sensation of fatigue, stop immediately and seek medical attention.

If you have had an event *(heart attack or problem such as heart failure or stroke):*

Have your doctor tailor your exercise program based on your clinical condition.

In general, we advocate:

- Be sure to warm up longer in order to prepare your cardiovascular system for the effort.
- Start with mild activity to give your cardiovascular system time to develop.
- Walk on flat surfaces to start with.
- At the beginning, exclude activity that works your upper body, such as shoveling, lifting heavy weights, doing chin-ups. Activity that is concentrated in your upper extremities is a little more dangerous than milder activity that involves more of your total muscle mass.

If you have type 1 diabetes:

Aerobic activity is great for you—it burns sugar and increases your peripheral sensitivity to insulin. You may experience light-headedness as you begin to exercise. If you experience this—or any symptoms of low blood sugar—eat a little more before and during exercise. Continue to take your medication, but discuss with your doctor adjustments to your therapy as you grow your level fitness.

If you have high blood pressure:

Work on your endurance with mild- to moderate-intensity exercise, sustained for a long time. Choose an activity that employs a number of muscles in a very rhythmic pattern such as walking, riding a bike on the flats (at least in the beginning), cross-country skiing, in-line skating, swimming. All of these activities can reduce blood pressure in a significant percentage of people. Do *not* discontinue your medication. After you have established your exercise program, talk to your doctor again about the possibility of reducing your medication.

If you are a smoker:

The good news is that quitting smoking is the one thing that best reduces your overall risk of death—you have something non-smokers don't have! If you have lung limitations, or COPD, check with your doctor. Then start with aerobic activity at low intensity so the oxygen-carrying system can develop. (This will take time because it is limited by lung performance.) You can also use weights to increase your muscle mass. In particular, work to increase the strength of your core and respiratory muscles.

If you have a high BMI or hypertension:

Activities that are a good combination of aerobic and weight lifting (using light weight and high reps) offer the most benefit in burning fat, especially subabdominal fat. That's why adding weight lifting to any exercise program helps so much—it increases lean body mass and thus boosts metabolism. For activities that are purely aerobic, select those that are partially or non–weight bearing: moderate cycling, swimming, rowing, and so on. Avoid jogging, running, walking downhill, which can be very hard on your back and knees.

If you have a combination of the above risk factors, you need to talk to your doctor or come to see us: http://intermountainhealthcare.org

Find the Right Doctor

My father is a physician. If ever there were injuries, they got addressed right away. He was innovative with treatment options—he'd set a hockey player's broken wrist while he was holding a stick, for example, so it would be in the right position for him to play with the cast on. I broke my leg skating short track, and my father made a two-part long-leg cast so I could take off the top half to ride a bike and stay in shape.

—Eric

It can be difficult to find a health-care provider who offers good medical treatment with consideration for your fitness aspirations, especially when you have an injury. When you go to the doctor with a problem caused by your beloved activity, you don't want one who will simply say, "Well, don't do it anymore."

Most physicians in the United States are under tremendous pressure to see many patients a day, so they want to get you out of the door as quickly as possible. But rest assured that there *are* health-care providers out there who will sit down and listen to you and give you advice on dealing with your injury in a way that doesn't preempt your desire to stay active. Just keep asking around; it's worth it. Look for a doctor who's willing to work with your specific concerns and who will respect your desire to pursue your chosen activity.

In addition, you need to become educated about your health. When getting prescriptions, physical therapy, or treatments of any kind, or when considering surgery, you need to research available options and ask your doctor for the treatment best suited to your active life.

I wanted to do a favorite double century (a two-hundred-mile bike ride in a day) three months after knee reconstruction. I asked my surgeon.

"I'm not enthused about your driving so long without getting up and moving, but as long as the car isn't a manual transmission . . ."

He had trepidation about my *driving* two hundred miles. After my many reassurances (read: begging), he gave me the green light.

I asked more questions when selecting doctors after that.

Years later, when I was pregnant and wanted to do another double century or, say, a 2,500-foot rock climb, I asked my OB/GYN, herself an avid rower. She wasn't shocked and overcautious.

"You've done this before, right?" she'd ask. "Then stay hydrated and have fun."

—DeAnne

ACUTE INJURIES

Even with the right gear and best form, injuries do happen. Here are a few of the most common and how you or a health-care provider might treat them.

Abrasions

One of the most common injuries in almost any activity is abrasions. To treat one:

1. Clean the abrasion well. It's best to get in the shower and clean it with a soft surgical scrub brush and ordinary antibacterial soap. Make an effort to remove all dirt, gravel, and grease. Any debris left in the wound will leave a tattoo on your skin.
2. Dress the wound. Abrasions require a special dressing. The gold standard is bioclusive dressings, but you can also use nonadhesive or Vaseline-impregnated gauze, which is about one-tenth the cost of a bioclusive.
3. If you don't mind higher cost and maintenance, bioclusive dressings afford a greater degree of moist-wound protection. They keep abrasions clean and dry, much like a Gore-Tex bandage might. They let fluid out and nothing in. But they are not cheap, must be changed every couple of days, and need to be ordered online. Apply a bioclusive after the wound has been cleaned out, and it will dry to the wound like a scab. Simply use scissors to trim any raised edges.

Acute Strain

An acute strain occurs when a muscle or tendon is stretched or torn. If this happens you will notice immediate pain, tenderness, and swelling. You may never experience an acute strain—most active people do not—but if you do, it's something you can treat at home:

1. Apply ice to the area.
2. Take an antiinflammatory as directed.
3. After any acute soreness is relieved, start a stretching program. Stretch up to and just before the point at which you would make the area sore.
4. Resume activity gradually.
5. Give it time to heal.

Meniscus Tear

The meniscus is a crescent-shaped cartilage pad in your knee joint that provides a smooth surface on which your femur and tibia move. When you're young it's spongy and resilient, but as you age it becomes brittle and fragile, like rubber that's been left out in the sun. You can tear it just by squatting to pick up the newspaper.

The meniscus is injured most often during exercise when the knee is rotated while bearing weight, for example, in basketball, volleyball, skiing, skating, football, and soccer—sports where you are required to cut or pivot.

If you tear a meniscus, your symptoms will be knee pain with a catching or grinding sensation; your knee might even lock up and not move fully. Also, there will be some swelling with activity. If this occurs, you should:

1. Avoid the activities that cause the symptoms for a week or two.
2. If symptoms continue after a short period of rest, seek medical advice.
3. If your knee locks, seek medical attention within a few days.

What if I have scoliosis in my family? What exercise should I do?

Scoliosis, or curvature of the spine, can run in families and is seen more often in women. A routine physical examination should include screening for scoliosis. If scoliosis is detected, then pursue expert medical advice and have it followed in case there is progression of the curve. Meanwhile, concentrate on low-back and core exercise.

What if I've been told I might have exercise-induced asthma?

Exercise-induced asthma is mild, exercise-induced bronchial spasms or asthma, but many people aren't even aware that they have it. The symptoms of exercise-induced mild asthma are not obvious. They include:

- coughing during warm-up or cool-down periods
- the sensation of shortness of breath with cold or polluted air
- breathing that is cut short

If these symptoms bother you or affect the quality of your workout, you should speak to your doctor regarding asthma. You should also avoid starting any workout too quickly in dry, cold, or polluted air, particularly when dehydrated. One of the triggering factors of exercise-induced asthma is dehydration, which causes coughing. That extra air you breathe dries out airways, and their receptors get hypersensitive.

You may need longer warm-ups to ready your muscles. If all of your muscles and organs (heart and lungs) are prepared when you begin your workout, you will not need to breathe as deeply or as often. If you start slowly enough, you can exercise through asthma.

If breathing problems make you quit workouts or cause you to lag behind your workout partners, it's worth talking to your doctor. Simple medication, modified warm-up methods, and breathing exercises and techniques to strengthen the respiratory muscles may be all you need for mild asthma. You don't cure your asthma, but you can move up your threshold. Rarely do people with mild asthma require an inhaler; their lung function in resting condition is normal.

In the 1980s I was working with a cyclist who was an under-achiever. She had potential, but for some reason she was never at her best. In particular, she had trouble at the beginning of the race, but she was one of the strongest at the end. We sent her to the pulmonology lab and found she had exercise-induced bronchial spasms (asthma). We started treatment with medication, and she went on to win a medal at the world championship.

—Max

What if my doctor tells me I'm anemic?

A good number of athletes face this when they start exercising. When you have a blood test, a lab counts the number of red blood cells in 100 milliliters of blood. Because exercise increases the plasma to a greater ratio than it increases the red blood cells, the red cell count appears low or in the anemic range. This is called pseudo-anemia because it's not really anemia; people who exercise generally have more than enough red blood cells. If the lab were to measure the person's overall quantity of blood, the lab would see the person has more blood and greater hemoglobin mass than the average person.

What if I have osteoporosis or it runs in my family?

Every woman needs to do weight-bearing activity, but particularly if you have osteoporosis or osteopenia, or if osteoporosis runs in your family. Weight-bearing activity includes walking and running, which have impact, which improves bone growth. In fact, any activity that has impact will increase bone growth—jump rope, trampoline, dance, and so on. Swimming is too low impact, and some say cycling is, too. (Studies show that bone density is lower in cyclists.) Others say cycling is good because it's gentler on those who already have osteoporosis. An elliptical trainer is also gentler than running but includes some weight-bearing mechanisms, so it helps increase bone growth.

What if there simply are not enough hours in the day to get everything done *and* a workout?

Try combining exercise with something you currently do. You may even *gain* some time. If you usually drive the kids to school or friends' houses, bike or walk with them instead. Driving there may take twenty-five minutes, riding bikes thirty-five—so a thirty-five-minute workout only "costs" you an additional ten minutes. Do yard work or housework at an aerobic pace. Seize every opportunity you are given to lift, walk, move, and carry. Or try workouts with a good time-to-benefit ratio, such as:

- interval training
- running
- mountain biking (which offers a good overall workout in a shorter amount of time than regular cycling)

What if I plan to work out but something always seems to come up?

If you frequently break your workout dates with yourself—something comes up, someone needs you, things tend to take priority over your workout—joining a group can be very motivating. You will have a set time at which everyone meets. That's more like an appointment, and you'll be less likely to break it. People will be counting on you to show up.

The social aspect is also very appealing, so you will be even more en-thused about going. And a group can be like a "workout community" where you can share information, ask questions, get insight from old-timers, and more.

What if I take so long to get dressed and get my gear together, I don't have any time left to exercise?

Get everything ready in advance. Check your bike tires. Fill your water bottle. Have your cycling or running or gym clothes, socks, helmet, sunglasses, and shoes—whatever you need—ready and in one place. Streamline your routine for getting out the door. Also, choose an activity that optimizes your time. For instance, running for thirty minutes is the equivalent of cycling for two hours, and you start getting the benefits of running right away. On the bike, you're a half hour into the ride before you start to benefit. Swimming for twenty minutes gives your body the same aerobic workout as walking for thirty-five. Jumping rope for three minutes is the equivalent of jogging for a half hour or playing tennis for an hour.

"How idiotic civilization is! Why be given a body if you have to keep it shut up in a case like a rare fiddle?"

—Katherine Mansfield

9
better cross-training

When I was skating, we skated outside and there was ice for only a fraction of the year. So we would have to do a lot of other cross-training type things to stay in shape. That's how I got into cycling. We used to lift weights a couple of times a week. We did a lot of running. I enjoyed all of them, and I also enjoyed the sheer variety. I certainly wouldn't want to do one all the time, but to have the variety and the camaraderie with my teammates was a lot of fun.

—Eric

Cross-training is using any type of exercise outside your primary sport to help you stay—or become more—fit. You will want to cross-train under a variety of circumstances: out of season, when you're just starting out, when injured or away from your specific sport, to maximize weight loss, or in extreme weather.

The classic goal of cross-training is to use multiple types of exercise so that the fatigue of a single muscle group or unfriendly weather doesn't stop you from working your cardiovascular system and other muscle groups. You can also use cross-training if you have an injury that keeps you from your usual activity. Cross-training allows you to stress your heart and lungs without stressing the injury. It also works well when you want to lose weight and when you're just starting out, by allowing you to continue exercising when you might otherwise be tired.

Why Cross-Train

You can use cross-training during your primary sport's off-season, when you are injured and unable to do your sport, or when weather does not permit you to do your sport. This can improve your fitness in two different ways. It can expand your aerobic foundation. Or it can develop specific qualities that you can later transfer to your primary activity.

I discovered running through Allan Claremont, an exercise physiologist at the Madison Speed Skating Club. When I was fifteen we also did cycling, mostly as cross-training for skating. The crossover [the physical requirements] of skating and cycling was close, and since there were no covered rinks, cycling allowed us to train in summer. I started racing a bit and found I really enjoyed it.

—Eric

The first goal of most cross-training programs is to concentrate solely on building a strong foundation by boosting your body's basic systems: heart, lungs, circulation, and muscles. This creates a very strong, wide base to support the pyramid of skills specific to your sport that you will develop later when you can do it again. Remember, the wider your base of aerobic and muscular ability, the taller your skill pyramid can go.

You can also cross-train to hone facets of skills specific to your activity. In other words, you can focus on one pinpointed adaptation that will contribute to bettering a single component of your sport. You might do plyometrics, for example, to improve your explosive movements in soccer, basketball, dance, or volleyball.

Cross-training is also very effective in keeping you in the groove. Once you have developed the habit of exercise, like an elite athlete you will very rarely want to do long periods of total rest when injured, off-season, or during inclement weather. Athletes often fear they will lose the training benefits that they've worked so hard to gain. If you feel this way, you won't feel good on total rest.

Here are some suggestions for appropriate cross-training modalities while healing from injury and in other circumstances:

■ If your sport is running, you might cross-train using cycling, cross-country skiing, hiking, skating, even martial arts.

- If you develop knee pain doing running, soccer, basketball, or aerobic dance, you could cross-train without pain in most cases riding a bike.
- People with Achilles tendonitis can often do aqua jogging or swimming (without kicking, using the breaststroke, for example).
- If you are a rower or tennis player with an elbow or wrist injury, you can run or ride a bike.
- If you want to lift weights but have back pain, instead of free weights you might use weight machines. These are a little easier on your back. Or instead of squatting with a barbell on your shoulder, you can use a leg press.
- If you sprain your ankle, you might run in water or ride a bike while you are recovering (stabilize your ankle if you do the latter).
- If you have shoulder pain, you can use your legs to get your heart and lungs working, by running, or using a StairMaster, for example.
- "Active rest," such as stretching, works for a day or two off from any other activity.
- When it's too hot or too cold outdoors, the gym is ideal. You can use any of the ergometers (treadmill, cyclette, rowing machines, or Stair-Master) and weight lifting.

When Cross-Training Doesn't Work

The downside to cross-training is that you lose specificity. For instance, if you're a good runner and use swimming to cross-train, you won't get much better at running. Say an athlete has the goal of running a faster marathon. So she runs two days a week, lifts weights at the gym for a half hour a day, and takes a Spinning class and two aerobic dance classes on weekends. And then she gives up because her running isn't getting any better. This, believe it or not, is classic. To get better at a sport, it's *better to do the sport*. If you want to win the Tour de France, sooner or later you better ride the bike. Sometimes you can't do your sport, however, and that's when cross-training is advisable.

Improper cross-training (cross-training in a sport that does not complement the sport you want to excel in) can also send your body contradictory signals. If you want to become a marathoner, for example, you don't want to lift weights like a bodybuilder, because as you get bigger and heavier with bodybuilding, you will develop muscles you won't need as a marathoner—but you will still have to carry them on your runs. And those muscles you develop can actually diminish your body's ability to develop the muscular qualities you *do* need as a marathoner.

Likewise, if you build maximum strength by using heavy weights with a low number of repetitions, you are doing excellent exercise for developing fast-twitch muscle fibers (see Chapter 2, where we go into your different muscle fibers in greater detail). Great—unless your goal is cycling, a sport that doesn't require maximum strength but instead requires a lot of oxygen going to the muscle fibers, preferably *slow-twitch* fibers. If you're a cyclist looking to improve climbing or time trialing, or a marathoner, you do not want to spend a lot of time developing the fast-twitch fibers of a bodybuilder, because these consume oxygen that would otherwise go to the small, slow-twitch fibers that push you in a marathon or on Alpe d'Huez. The fast-twitch fibers of bodybuilders and sprinters are also big in size, increasing the distance between the blood (and the oxygen) and the mitochondria, your energy plants.

Basic cross-training guidelines:

- If you want to maintain strength for an explosive sport, such as basketball, volleyball, or soccer, don't cross-train doing a lot of aerobic work. You may lose explosive strength as you transform some of the fast-twitch fibers to slow-twitch.
- If you are a light, endurance athlete, don't cross-train doing a lot of bodybuilding, because the bulk may work against you in your chief sport. Instead, use resistance training to make your muscles stronger and more resistant to fatigue.

Cross-Training for Weight Loss or When Just Starting Out

Cross-training is a great strategy for making the most of your workouts, either when just starting out and you tire easily or when you want to go longer than you normally could so that you can burn more calories. You will be able to do, for example, ten minutes each on a stair climber, a treadmill, and an elliptical trainer whereas it might be impossible to do thirty minutes on just one machine.

When you cross-train in these instances, you will want to combine several activities so that you can exercise longer than you could doing one activity continuously. In this way, you will not be limited by the localized fatigue of one muscle or a group of muscles. You can switch activities, go longer, and burn more calories or boost your aerobic training.

Cross-Training When Injured

Another major purpose of cross-training is to span an injury-imposed gap in your favorite activity. While an acute injury is healing, cross-training allows you to maintain your aerobic fitness. We also have patients who find that they have to abandon an activity altogether because they have a degenerative disease and a joint is slowly deteriorating. They need to find a completely different activity to engage in permanently, an activity that doesn't impact the affected joint. The tips we recommend for cross-training during injury are also helpful in these instances.

For knee problems, select activities that are non–weight bearing or only partially weight bearing, such as:

- Swimming
- Cycling (with a correct bike fit, on flat roads, using high cadence and a small gear to reduce the stress on your knees; also consider shortening the crank arms)
- Spinning
- Walking on a treadmill
- Aqua jogging (particularly if the injury is temporary)

Avoid:

- Jogging or running

For shoulder issues, try:

- Cycling
- Walking
- Jogging or running

Avoid:

- Swimming
- Racquet sports
- Golf
- Any activity that triggers symptoms

For Achilles tendon trouble, consider:

- Aqua jogging (if you got your injury running uphill)
- Swimming, ideally using breaststroke (don't use fins, and don't push off the pool wall)
- Cycling (see precautions, below)
- In-line skating (with your foot immobilized in the boot)

   Avoid:

- The activity that triggered the problem
- Running fast or running uphill
- If cycling, avoid: sprinting, frequently standing on your toes, climbing, or a bike-shoe cleat position that's too far forward or a bike-saddle position that's so high you have to point your toes

For a wrist injury, you may use:

- Jogging or running
- Hiking uphill
- Snowshoeing
- Ice skating or in-line skating (wear wrist protection)
- Cycling (with a good bike fit and high-quality grips on the handlebars, possibly aerobars)

   Avoid:

- Tennis
- Rowing
- Swim strokes that cause symptoms
- Cross-country skiing
- Walking on your hands (just kidding . . .)

For back pain, get assessed by your physical therapist or physician. Loss of strength, in particular, but also numbness are big red flags. If allowed by your health-care provider, consider:

- Pilates or yoga (at the right level) to strengthen your core muscles
- Swimming (avoid breaststroke, backstroke, butterfly)

■ Cycling, if your back pain comes from running. If your back pain was caused by cycling, get a bike fit.

Cross-Training to Peak

Cross-training can also be used to put you in the best possible condition for a specific week or event. This is referred to as cross-training to peak.

Does your goal include a date or a time frame? Do you want to compete in or complete an event or benefit, or prepare for an active vacation or a seasonal team sport? Then you want to plan to peak. Approaching a marathon, for example, you could ride a bike a couple of times a week, instead of running. This will allow your muscles to recover while you continue to somewhat stress your cardiovascular system. Be sure to avoid big, heavy gears; you want to keep your muscles supple on the bike.

Tapering is another method you can employ in order to peak. (For more on tapering to peak, see Chapter 7.)

10

better motivation

In our lifelong interest in exercise, we have learned some things through our education and through experience. One of the things we recognize is that there are areas where we do not know much. When we are asked questions in those areas, we always turn to people who are expert in that field.

One of the experts we rely on regarding questions of sports motivation is Eric's longtime friend Michael Lardon, M.D., associate professor at the University of California at San Diego, psychiatrist for the PGA Tour and the Olympics, and author of *Finding Your Zone: Ten Core Lessons for Achieving Peak Performance in Sports and Life.*

As a psychiatrist, Dr. Lardon has thought a great deal about human motivation on a scientific and a medical level. How do you get motivated? How do you stay motivated? And how do you avoid the pitfalls of losing your drive? Everyone needs the answers to these questions as they pursue fitness.

The Biology of Motivation

There is actually a biological component to motivation: Your body experiences a change physiologically when you are inspired. Think that your thoughts don't cause a biological reaction in your body? Have you ever witnessed something that made you physically ill? Positive thoughts have an equally strong but *positive* effect.

Such neurobiological rewards are in fact twofold. The natural endorphins your body releases when you exercise are well known. These endorphins are basically natural opiates that live in your body. You activate them when you exercise, and as a result you experience a sort of high. But another natural reward system that resides within your body is far more significant than endorphins, and that is dopamine.

Dopamine is a neurotransmitter within your brain. When people take drugs such as cocaine or methamphetamine, it prompts the release of dopamine. Nicotine also releases dopamine—that's why it's so hard to quit smoking. When a boy hits a home run in a Little League game and you watch him run around the bases, dopamine is released in your brain. When you fall in love, dopamine is released. All of these things engage what is called the dopamine reward pathway. In other words, you are rewarded with dopamine when you have these experiences, and the sensation derived is so pleasurable that you become driven to experience them again.

The dopamine response system is powerfully motivating. In experiments with rats that can choose either cocaine or food, the rats will choose the cocaine again and again until they've starved to death. That's a staggering amount of motivation.

Exercise also releases dopamine. That first week of exercise is hard to start, but once you engage the dopamine reward pathway, your body becomes unconsciously driven to experience more exercise. This motivation can overcome almost any level of inertia. Have you ever seen someone out for a jog, in driving rain, in the dark? What you are very likely seeing is the potent dopamine reward pathway in action.

The feel-good response of the dopamine reward pathway is much more all-encompassing than simply the "runner's high," which is based merely on endorphins. You might not even reach a runner's high if you use a treadmill for twenty minutes; the endorphin system takes longer than twenty minutes to kick in. But when you're starting out and you use the treadmill for twenty minutes, you *definitely* engage the dopamine reward pathway. You will feel really good about yourself, even after the first time, before the association is firmly established. And once it is established, that association will be reinforced every time you exercise and experience the exhilaration once again. Soon exercise becomes something you look forward to: Exercise itself becomes a reward.

Motivation and Action

There are conscious ways of motivating yourself as well. According to Dr. Lardon, motivation is goal oriented. Having a goal is a way you activate your behavior with a purpose and a direction. You might have all sorts of high emotions and desires, constantly thinking, I want to do this, I want to do that, but very few people can channel that into action. When you can, that emotion is called motivation.

Putting emotion to work in this way is not mind-over-matter, or chanting mantras "I *will* work out, I *will* work out." As physicians, not one of the three of us would espouse such chicanery. We are scientists, so we are neither optimists nor pessimists, we are realists. Dr. Lardon's approach to harnessing your emotion to create motivation has been proven effective in studies and it utilizes the *truth* about your athletic experiences.

It starts with the simplest of tools: your self-confidence. Self-confidence is one of your most basic needs, according to Abraham Maslow. In his famous *Hierarchy of Needs in Human Beings*, Maslow lists competence and self-actualization as a human's highest need. This leader in the humanistic school of psychology in the fifties and sixties delineated four levels in the hierarchy of needs in human beings. The most basic concerns the need for food, water, and shelter. Next, come safety and security. The third level is family, friends, and feeling accepted. And the highest level is competence and self-actualization. Dr. Lardon believes that these basic needs fuel your motivation in everything you do, from exercise to the dishes.

Before winning the world speed-skating championships for the first time, I was fortunate enough to receive a letter from my coach. She was unable to attend, but said that I should have confidence in my ability. She wrote: "Don't be satisfied with second best." That got me over the psychological edge my competitor had on me.

—Eric

Gauge Small Improvements Objectively

No one resents the most basic scientific facts. You don't talk about the unfairness of gravity or the favoritism of physics. Yet as people coach themselves through exercise, they may react to what seems like the general unfairness of it all. A lot of questions we get are about just that: "Why is this person better than me?" For the answer, we tell them to look to the science of exercise. Just as we respect physics, we must also respect the laws of exercise: the roles of genetics, training, biological adaptation, periodization, motivation, and so on. These, too, are scientific fact.

As a good self-coach, you will need to use intelligence and mental focus to recognize and compensate for any gap you might have in physical ability. To do so, you need to arm yourself with the laws of training science. One of the best ways to stay away from self-criticism and keep the spotlight on progress is by gauging small improvements objectively via testing: self-testing, field testing, lab testing, measuring your abilities at the beginning of your training and all along the way—something very few programs talk about. (See Chapter 2 regarding gauging small improvements, and Part Two for detailed testing instructions.) This way, you turn your attention toward objective data and away from subjective opinion, yours or anyone else's.

Pinpoint Your Inner and Outer Sources

There are various sources of motivation, and you as an individual derive your motivation from different things than anyone else might. Dr. Lardon has written about the two general types of motivation: extrinsic and intrinsic. Intrinsic or inner motivations have to do with exploring your own abilities, for enjoyment, health, or self-actualization. Intrinsic satisfaction might come from shaving two seconds off your time, sticking with your exercise program, or moving in small, preset increments toward your goal of doing a 10k run—all the things for which you will pat yourself on the back. Intrinsic motivation is the desire to explore your own personal limits, to see what you're made of.

Extrinsic or outer motivations are derived from sources outside yourself: attention, praise, applause, placing at a certain level in competition, fame and fortune, or social reinforcement. The former are easy to recognize; the latter, social reinforcement, could include running because you do it with a group of people you like, or showing up at aerobics dance class because you are close to the regulars there. If you do the same run that shaves two seconds off your time, but the real goal is to beat your buddy, you're extrinsically motivated.

These inner and outer motivations drive you to your goals, and with each goal achieved, you will obtain greater self-esteem.

Keep Your Motivations Current

Dr. Lardon works primarily with golfers, professional ballplayers, and Olympic athletes, but his examples are universally instructive in how to stay motivated. One of his clients, for example, is the elite golfer Rich Beem. Rich beat Tiger Woods to win his first major, the 2002 PGA Championship.

But when Rich Beem started out, his motivations were not fame and fortune. Instead, he first played golf for fun. At the elite college level, his motivation changed and he was then driven to play golf to gain the respect of his peers. When he came into the pros, his motivation evolved to playing golf to make a good living. What drives him now is exploring his own abilities. But it took time and thought for him to arrive at this, once he had achieved a certain level of success.

"After Rich won the PGA Championship, he was bombarded with people and sponsors usurping his time. Like any elite athlete, it was easy for him to lose some focus and motivation," says Dr. Lardon. "Over the years we've talked many times and he has realized that fortune and fame is a by-product of his hard work and focus and if he still wants to improve he has to play for himself—play to explore his God-given gift. Rich has worked very hard the last few years and is once again centered. I would not be surprised if Beemer wins another major. He is a great champion and now his motivation is pure."

When you try to stay motivated to exercise, especially after you make it over that first little hump of success, you, too, may need to recalibrate, to lock on to something that is motivating to you *now*. You also need to understand that your motivation may continue to evolve over time. Let your motivation be dynamic.

Minimize Outside Stresses

If you really want to do well in a 10k run or a cycling race or in getting to the gym every afternoon, part of preparing for that is to make certain that most of your life is in order, or in the best order it can be. This allows you to channel your energy into the task at hand.

Jack Nicklaus won sixty golf tournaments and twenty majors altogether—more majors than anyone in history. But just like the rest of us, Jack now and then had problems with motivation. Before Jack could perform well at a golf tournament, he had to have his life in order. If he had a personal problem going on, say, at home or in his business, he would not golf as well as he wanted. In life, you can't always arrange everything to go perfectly, but Jack would at least try. Four times a year, when each of the major tournaments took place, he would do everything he could to bring order to his personal life. Dr. Lardon finds this works for others as well. So when you find yourself closing in on a specific exercise goal, don't pile on unnecessary additional social, family, and work obligations and stressors; being overburdened could cause defeat in the athletic arena.

Avoid Extreme Challenges

Another interesting theory of Dr. Lardon's has to do with the need for mental peace. Research has shown that many of us possess a need for being in a peaceful state. And if you are able to put yourself in a peaceful state, this will feed into what Mike calls "the flow and peak-experience phenomenon."

He explains: "When I was in college, I used to ride bikes with Eric and other great riders, these super-high-level guys, and I was just a regular guy. That was not a peaceful place for me. In fact, I would have tremendous anxiety."

Does anxiety improve your performance? You do the math. Part of your motivation is derived from matching your skill level with a task that's doable. People like to stretch a little bit, but if you put yourself in a situation that's extremely stressful—say, you try to do a triathlon that is way beyond your ability or your training—you aren't going to be encouraged by the experience and this will hamper your motivation.

So look for opportunities to stretch yourself a little. This can be motivating. But avoid putting yourself in a situation where you have very little probability of success. If you push yourself too hard or fast, the experience is only going to diminish your self-confidence and thus your motivation.

Easy Doesn't Do It

I trained hard and put in the time and effort. I didn't cut any corners.

—Eric

However, don't select goals that are too easy. If you're not creating a little bit of a stretch with your exercise, your brain loses interest. Your brain is an organ that, like a muscle, craves challenge. Dr. Lardon likens it to the requirement that medical students study calculus. "It's not like you are going to use the arithmetic tools of calculus in the practice of medicine," he says. "But the university makes medical students do it because it stretches your mind. It makes your mind think in ways that it doesn't normally think."

There is motivation to be culled from experiences that challenge you. If you have a sense that you could do something that might stretch your limits and you decide to do it as an experience to stretch your limits (rather than to prevail), that practice will actually serve to *reinforce* your motivation. This is called a positive feedback cycle: You become more motivated when you think there's a greater probability of success. Putting yourself in situations where you might triumph, or where you think that you can at least handle it, increases your motivation. And the more you think there's a possibility of success, the more motivated you become.

Recharging Self-Confidence

Stretching yourself a little bit fulfills your need to feel competent and have a sense of control. It all comes back to your self-esteem, according to Dr. Lardon. And through the scientific research that's been done on the topic, self-confidence has proven very, *very* important for anyone who plans to stay motivated in their own exercise program. You can recharge your self-confidence with thoughts from three basic domains.

Modeling Somebody Else's Behavior

You obtain self-confidence via modeling someone else's behavior when you watch someone do something, observe how they do it, and then decide that you can do it, too, by copying their technique. You watch a videotape of a skier with perfect form, and the next time you go skiing you imitate his behavior. A good example outside of sports is the story Oprah Winfrey tells about starting out her career in television imitating Barbara Walters's interviewing style. Oprah was certain that Barbara had it right, so she knew if she did what Barbara did, she would get it right. This increased her self-confidence when she went on the air.

Your Past Experiences

Your past experiences bestow confidence by becoming little coaches cheering in your head, You can do it! And you know with absolute certainty that you *can* because you think of experiences where you actually have done it.

Dr. Lardon recalls a time when his best friend Tommy, who plays at the local public golf course and has won the local championship a few times, called the night before one of the championships, anxious about the next day. To motivate Tommy, Dr. Lardon focused on building Tommy's self-confidence by recalling Tommy's past experiences. Dr. Lardon pointed out that Tommy had won the same championship four years ago, so obviously he could do it.

Recalling past experiences is the most effective of the three domains because it is the most data driven. When using this technique, think about your past experiences doing similar things, and pull out your *best* past experiences. Those are true data points: when you had your best run, best ride, or best exercise session. Don't focus on the time you had a terrible run, lost, flailed, or left early. You focus on the best you have done because that *most honestly speaks to your true capacity.*

Vicarious Learning

You also gain self-confidence via vicarious learning, when you can say to yourself, Well, she did it, and if she can do it, I can do it. It's success by association. Dr. Lardon offers another example from Rich Beem's success:

"We've already talked about Rich Beem. When he was in college, he had known two college friends who continued to pursue professional golfing careers. After a time, Rich had quit golf, but soon thereafter both his friends went on to win on the PGA Tour. When word reached Beem of his buddies' success, Beem was selling cell phones in Seattle for about $15 an hour. He thought, Geez, Louise, if they can do it, and I can beat them I can do it, too. Rich decided to go give professional golf another try and the rest is history." This is a great example of how vicarious learning can lead to building self-confidence.

Focus Trumps Talent

There are many people who are talented at various athletic activities, yet what differentiates those who most successfully pursue athletics from those who don't is what Dr. Lardon calls "this thing between the ears: your brain." Your brain provides mental focus. There are people with great physical ability who never cultivate their focus and as a result they don't explore their true potential.

Good examples of people with great ability but no focus are professional athletes who are very inconsistent, people, Dr. Lardon says, who "have all the talent in the world, and they're all over the place."

People who are successful time and again—the ones who keep going—are those who have harnessed the tremendous power of data (the reality of their athletic experiences) and the ability of their brain to focus and motivate themselves. It's very unusual to see those things mated. Jack Nicklaus had it; Tigers Woods has it. The Tigers and the Jacks have incredible mental focus, as well as stellar physical ability. Michael Jordan had it, too. But Dr. Lardon points out that Jordan barely made his college basketball team. Which demonstrates that when you want to give up based on what might be perceived as failure on a physical level, your brain has to kick in and utilize effective motivational tools to span the gap, to keep you going and doing well until you experience the next success. In fact, as you move up the performance ladder and get better and better, the more mental focus is going to matter.

The Gift of the Present

One of the ways to continue successfully after what might be perceived as failure is by cultivating the mental discipline of staying in the present.

"You do your best when there's only one shot, one ride, one run on your mind: the next one," says Dr. Lardon. If you worry about your last performance or about what's going to happen in the future, you might want to stay home and hide in a closet.

Imagine being a professional athlete and making a terrible shot in front of a crowd. Most people would be embarrassed. But the best professional athletes just aren't. They call upon their unbelievable focus and motivation to be in the present and execute the *next* shot with just as much full commitment, as if nothing has happened, regardless of the context. Dr. Lardon calls this decontextualization. He applies the term to an athlete's ability to perform the same way whether in front of huge crowds or by herself, even after she has goofed up.

Dr. Lardon points out that if you can decontextualize, you don't care about the past. You don't care if you were never an athlete in high school—you're going to exercise. You don't care if you can't dance—you are going to take an aerobic dance class. You don't care if you failed the last ten times you started an exercise program—you only care about the one you're starting now. You don't care about embarrassment or what people think; the "you should be this, you should be that" kind of thing is irrelevant. You leave aside how you're perceived. Concentrating on the negative things other people might think eats away at your motivation, and it's really none of your concern anyway, Dr. Lardon points out. This is harder, of course, if your motivation is derived from accolades, but it's easy if you are exercising for inner rewards, such as improving yourself, your health, your weight, your time, or your longevity.

When I was younger, I had a daily goal of doing well at whatever I was training that day, and if I didn't, the next day I had to make up for the intensity I missed. My daily reward was the feeling of having gotten through a workout and done it well. If I was running quarter miles at race pace, I ran *every one* at race pace. My daily goal was not to cheat myself.

—Eric

Dr. Lardon cites Eric as an example of an athlete who is able to decontextualize. "It doesn't matter to Eric if he's alone with his buddies or in front of millions of people. That's egoless motivation—he's enjoying it. For him it's about self-exploration, not about what anyone thinks."

The Misfortune of Believing in "Luck"

Many of the people we see mention luck with regard to their exercise program in their early visits. They seem to believe that whether or not they accomplish their exercise goal comes down to luck. Let's just say that they are soon cured of this misperception.

Dr. Lardon calls a belief in luck attribution. If you believe your success is simply a matter of luck and that you don't have any control over the situation, this is an external attribution: You are handing over control of the outcome to something outside of yourself, something external.

This can occur when you tell yourself that certain situations or items are necessary for you to succeed, or when you tell yourself, It's a bad course for me, or I don't like running on rainy days, or I've had a bad day at work, and it's only going to get worse if I go to yoga tonight. Whether you think you're having bad luck or good, essentially it is the same: You are telling yourself that you have no control, that *you* can't do it. Ultimately, a belief in luck takes the power out of your hands and erodes your motivation.

Instead, take control over your performance. Acknowledge that your fitness success is not a matter of luck. If things seem to be going badly, reinforce your confidence by noting factors that *are* in your favor and you will regain control. For example, ignore the rain or the bad day and tell yourself, I've trained really hard, I'm ready to go, and I feel I can do it. Doing this is intrinsic or internal attribution. These kinds of statements firmly and confidently put the power in your own hands and build up your self-confidence and motivation.

[At the Lake Placid Olympics] the night before the 10,000-meter speed-skating race, the United States played Russia in hockey. I'm an avid hockey fan and I grew up in Madison playing hockey with a couple of the guys on the team—Mark Johnson and Bobby Suter. I had only missed one of their games. After watching the Russia/USA hockey game, we all walked out of there with big smiles on our faces.

That night I was certainly fatigued from the previous races, but I think staying up late watching that game also caught up with me in the end. The following morning, I overslept. I woke up to my coach pounding on my door. I grabbed a slice of bread for breakfast, and barely made it to the rink in time for my race.

My routine was normally to get to the rink two hours before a race, but not this time. I realized what I had to do to accomplish what I wanted. I couldn't think about oversleeping, not eating breakfast, not getting my usual routine at the rink. I had to just concentrate on what was in front of me.

—Eric

Despite all of these factors that Eric could have perceived as bad luck, he won the gold medal in the 10,000-meter race and set a world record.

When you feel you have control, you discover you *can* control what happens to you by simply doing what you do as well as you can. According to Dr. Lardon, when you think you can control what you're trying to do, it truly makes a difference. Suddenly it becomes *your* exercise program, *your* workout, *your* time to take care of *your*self. And you wouldn't let anyone take it away from you.

Avoid Blame

There are other types of negative external attribution, such as blame and unnecessary self-consciousness, both of which are equally detrimental to your motivation.

You may have ability, yet still waste your time to exercise because of your perception of what other people are thinking. Examples include such thoughts as, There's too much politics involved in that league, or the coach will never play me, and when he does he'll only put me up against the pitchers that I can't hit. This happens on community ball teams as well as in the major leagues. If you tell yourself, It's team politics, or the Pilates instructor is out to get me, you *are* going to do worse. Then you'll think, See? I knew it.

External attribution can also work against you if you are just starting out and hesitant to go to the gym, take a class, or join a team. You might think, People will stare or laugh at me, or those people aren't very friendly. In both cases, you will bolster your confidence if you instead think about what you *are* good at and what you *do* have control over: I'm a good hitter. I'm going to take a good swing, make good contact, and get a hit.

You need to take control of what happens to you—and, as we've said before, you do have a good deal of control. In this way, your goals will also shore up your courage. When you begin feeling governed by self-consciousness, turn your focus to your goals instead. Think: I can go to the gym today and do twenty minutes. This will do much more to reinforce your exercise habit than worrying about the hard-bodied guy next to you, or the neighbor who can go for an hour, or Eric who can go forever.

The Dual Reward of Rewards

Everyone needs a carrot—some kind of reward you are chasing along with your goal. For many people, just making it to the end of a workout is enough of a reward, but other rewards are necessary, too. Part of the reason professional athletes are so motivated is that they receive multiple rewards for doing well, from sponsors, from coaches, from the public, as well as from themselves. You don't get any of those, so it's doubly important that you find ways to reward yourself when you exercise. Rewards need not cost money. A reward can be a weekend free from household chores, or time to hang out with a friend or read a book. In medical school, Dr. Lardon rewarded himself with basketball if he completed his studies each day. We have athletes who reward themselves with vacations after the season is over *only* if they accomplish their goal. We also know people who reward themselves with a nice evening out if they produce a good result.

It's not always enough to know that you'll feel better if you exercise. That helps, but for those days when it's not enough, the promise of a preset reward may be just enough to get you out the door. You're human—without a reward, you will find that some days you are going to come up empty, motivationwise. Dr. Lardon finds the reward strategy helps make people consistent.

I try to make sure I have two scheduled rides where people count on me and I count on them. It motivates me to have a workout partner or other people to exercise with. I'm motivated by the camaraderie, the culture, and the encouragement. When it comes to competition, I'm mostly looking at my physiological numbers—wattage, power, knowing my previous numbers, but working out with other people spurs me on—they push me.

—Eric

Other "carrots" or rewards that may contribute to your motivation:

- Have a training partner you won't want to let down, like your dog.
- Don't put your treadmill in front of a white wall—put it near a TV, or get a book holder and read your favorite magazine.
- Join a group.
- Take a bike ride to check out the houses or the view en route.
- Think about who and what you see on your daily walks, rather than the exercise itself.
- Add music to your exercise with an MP3 player.
- Use the exercise as a means to convey you somewhere you really want to go: bicycle to the coffee shop or the library.

Heads Up

I enjoy music or watching TV when warming up, but during the workout I find it distracting. I'm not able to focus on the physical sensations and gauge my effort.

—Eric

Most of us try to distract ourselves from our sensations while we exercise—with music or training buddies, new routines or beautiful scenery, TV or reading material. It's as if we don't want to be there when it happens. And, frankly, routine exercise *can* be boring.

Whatever you can do to make it more pleasurable is welcome (as long as it doesn't impair your safety). Also, you will want to remove your headphones at least now and then and take a few minutes to think about your sensations and measure them for your diary. (For more information, see Chapter 8, "Better Motion and Gear.")

The Math of Motivation

Recognize that you *are* human, and you are going to want to give up when your performance dips. That's natural. In the beginning, you may think a poor workout means you are not cut out for fitness. Very often, however, a drop in performance is due to a stressful workweek, a cold, or a sleepless night with a sick child. You have heard that exercise relieves stress: You get home from a hard day at work, throw on your exercise clothes, and decide you're going to redeem the day with a stellar workout. And you find you can hardly get to the corner. That's because physiologically, stress in all parts of your life (work, family, health, diet, and sleep) has a cumulative effect and impacts performance not just on a mental but on a *physical* level. When the sum total overwhelms your system, it is not a decree that you are unfit for fitness. None of us is unfit for exercise. Still, the doubts may creep in. When that happens, think about other stresses that may be draining your energy for exercise.

Compare Yourself Only to Yourself

As a self-coach, you should compare yourself only to yourself. It is enough to think about. What you think is your limit may not be your limit if you haven't tried all the options. You may not do so if you are focused "out there." To self-coach successfully you need knowledge and *you need to apply it*, and then you need to measure how you—and only you—are doing. To determine whether you are making progress, how someone else is doing is irrelevant. If someone else is better or worse, it's not about you. The program is about exercise, not competition. It doesn't matter what anyone else is doing.

Staying motivated is a difficult and dynamic process, even with the dramatically persuasive powers of dopamine and your thoughts. Dr. Lardon likens it to a flowering plant. You nurture it, you grow it, you cut it back. It's not a static thing. You have to be aware of that and give it everything you've got to keep it going. How to sustain motivation is a question for everyone regarding every task in life. Everything you do today is compelled by a variety of motivations. To keep exercise part of your life, you need to bring into play as many motivations as you can. Think about it as a process and then approach it from all angles, prune it, and nurture it.

What if I prefer to work out alone? I like the meditative aspects of exercising by myself, but I keep hearing that I should work out with others. What are the pros and cons?

Some athletes such as trail runners, swimmers, and others who do their workouts solo gain some benefit from the time alone. It's good to spend time alone so you can listen to your body. How does my knee really feel? How hard can I push myself? People get overwhelmed with all the electronic monitors for tracking their heart rate, their power, their cadence, their mileage, and so on. When they lose battery power, they have no inner gauge for how they are doing. They have no idea how they should feel. Working out solo allows you to listen to and get to know your body and its sensations, so you will know how you are doing.

The downside to working out alone is that it's hard to challenge yourself enough. Working out with other people can challenge you, but be aware it can also make it difficult to follow your own scheduled program or stick to certain training zones. People in groups tend to get competitive. Or everyone will start doing one person's program. Or the group collapses into one big social outing. But if you find a group with whom you can stick to your scheduled program, the camaraderie can be very motivating.

PART TWO

the
program

You're now equipped to move forward and design your exercise program—to start putting on miles and purring like that well-oiled machine.

Using scientific principles, you'll design a program for yourself that is twelve weeks in length, long enough for your deep physiological metamorphosis to take hold. The design will be individualized, based on your starting point, which you will assess to establish an azimuth toward your goal; then you will tailor your program to your particular strengths and needs.

With that information in hand, you'll be able to treat exercise like the powerful drug that it is—taking it at the right time, in the right amount and intensity, for the right duration, in addition to providing your hardworking body with adequate recovery days and weeks. You'll also supply yourself with the right fuel and fluids, as well as well-fitting gear and good technique. In addition, you will troubleshoot aches and pains early and enlist the help of a physician to be there when the need arises.

Along the way, you'll remain in tune with your body via an exercise diary and will remain flexible to necessary adjustments. At the end of this section, we provide information on how to make those adjustments. To keep you going, you'll enlist the biological power of positive but fact-based thought, to reinforce the dopamine reward pathway with frequent and rewarding activity, and to motivate yourself with a major goal, and smaller goals along the way. All of these will reinforce the patience you'll utilize to see you through to the vast changes exercise will bring, no matter your starting point.

Assessments

First, the test drive. To plot your journey from your current condition to your goals, you need to establish your starting point. You'll do this through a few tests that will determine your current fitness levels. Once you ascertain your starting point we will know where you need to focus your energy and what level of intensity will serve you best. Too many fitness-seekers begin a program without knowing their starting point, which wastes time and energy, and, ultimately, can cause a loss of motivation. Knowing your strengths and weaknesses helps guarantee you the fastest return and furnishes you with a dependable compass for achieving fitness success.

Start a notebook to keep track of the results and to begin your exercise diary. You will also need to copy the chart below. Here you will record and track your test scores. (You can photocopy it from this book or download a blank from our Web site: www.fasterbetterstronger.com)

Cardiovascular Risk Assessment

Before starting your assessments, let's determine your cardiovascular risk factors. Ultimately, regular exercise reduces these risk factors, such as elevated cholesterol and high blood pressure (both of which contribute to the development of heart disease). But before you begin to exer-

Cardiovascular Risk Score	Aerobic Fitness Score	Muscular Strength Score	Flexibility Score	Balance and Coordinaion Scores	BMI	1RM	VO$_2$ Max
Score Week 1				Foot-raise:			
Score Week 6				Foot-raise:			
Score Week 12				Foot-raise:			

cise you need to know where you stand with regard to these risk factors.

By starting this exercise program today, you could be adding healthy, happy years to your life; it may add even more if you are at risk for heart disease. However, while exercising, you put more stress on your body, so a condition that has remained asymptomatic may suddenly rear its head and become symptomatic, with life-threatening consequences. The probability of your having silent problems is even greater if you have been sedentary for a long time.

Thus, the risk far outweighs the hassle of checking beforehand. Find out before you start exercising and challenging your heart. We recommend that everyone—especially those who have been very inactive up until now—have a physical before beginning this or any program.

Be aware that a regular run-of-the-mill physical has limited ability to reveal your true condition or problems that would arise with the amplification of exercise. When being examined while sitting on an exam table in a doctor's cubicle, patients often have regular heart rate and rhythm, normal blood pressure, clear lungs, no wheezing, and so on. However, when Max rechecks these same patients using various tests to examine them through the magnifying lens of exercise, he sees their functions more vividly. A person who breathes normally during their annual physical may have asthma when she starts exercising and demands more of her body. Another person who has no problem supplying oxygen to his heart in a resting condition may, while exercising, show symptoms of one of his coronary arteries being partially plugged. His heart suddenly has to pump two to three times as much blood, but the affected coronary artery isn't allowing enough blood and oxygen to supply the part of the heart that is now working double time. Patients, generally males in their fifties and sixties, will say, "Sometimes during exercise I have chest discomfort. It's not my heart, maybe just a strained muscle. Sometimes it goes away after I warm up, so I can do my workout." Then we do a stress ECG and a heart condition shows up. The test takes only an extra fifteen minutes, but on average we catch something every month.

Though stress tests don't catch 100 percent of these problems, a stress test is a simple way to learn more about your heart and your fitness. You can do a stress test riding a bike or walking on a treadmill, whichever you prefer.

Athletes are lucky. They catch their problems at an earlier stage because the problems become symptomatic when they challenge themselves through exercise. Unfortunately, people who are sedentary may not have chest pain until the disease is more advanced.

In many parts of the world, testing of every child with an interest in sports is a given. In some areas of Europe, screening for heart disease, using an ECG, begins at age twelve. There is no such law in the United States, since the cost-benefit ratio of the screening is still open for discussion. Some children's sports programs require that athletes get a doctor's preparticipation evaluation note, but many times these visits are seen as a waste of time. Thus, many Americans reach adulthood having never been screened via a supervised exercise stress test. We tend to think that if someone is fine, they *are* fine. And that's true for the majority. But we know that about 2.5 sudden deaths per 100,000 young athletes occur every year. Over 50 percent of these are preventable through screening. The numbers are definitely small, but they are significant, especially if they involve someone close to you.

This is not meant to scare you, but to convey to you the importance of preparticipation screening. So before you begin an exercise program for the first time or when you plan to embark on a new program even if you have been fit in the past, we recommend that you discuss topics relevant to athletic screening with your doctor, including:

1. Your past medical history, with a focus on cardiovascular disease, high blood pressure, elevated cholesterol, diabetes, asthma or allergies, and musculoskeletal conditions.
2. Your family history for sudden death, coronary heart disease (especially in first-degree relatives below age fifty to fifty-five), stroke, hypertension, and diabetes.
3. Your social history for cigarette smoking, drug use, and exercise habits.
4. A review of your systems, with particular attention to exercise-related symptoms (fainting, light-headedness, shortness of breath, wheezing, chest pain or tightness, palpitations, headache, and so on).

We also recommend a general physical exam, starting with your height and weight in order to assess your BMI (the ratio between your weight and the square of your height; we also offer instructions for doing this later in this chapter), and including an accurate measurement of your blood pressure, ideally in resting condition and again after a short effort, like a step test, a handgrip test, or going up stairs.

Based on the findings, your doctor will determine if you need further tests, such as blood work, pulmonary function test (PFT), stress test, or more.

Knowing your risk factors can be very motivating, because proper exercise will help lower your risk significantly. If you belong to a high-risk category (for example, you are an overweight, sedentary male smoker, over forty-five, with high blood pressure whose family has a history of heart attacks), you are the perfect candidate for our program—you can get better, but you will need to see your doctor before you begin. Exercise could become a significant component of your life, but you will want to tailor your program to take your risk factors into account. After six or twelve weeks, when regular, moderate-intensity exercise has brought down your risk for heart disease by lowering your cholesterol and/or blood pressure, you can then reevaluate your exercise intensity and plan a new program with your doctor's help.

If you have muscle issues (such as recurrent back pain, numbness in one leg when you walk, sciatica, or an unstable knee), you will also want to talk to your doctor.

Once you know your starting risk factors, you can use this information to evaluate your improvements. Having a risk factor does not preclude you from exercise—it simply requires more precise tailoring with the help of a personal physician, who will factor your risk into the equation when designing the intensity of your program.

Cardiovascular Risk Factors Test

The main risk in exercise comes from cardiovascular problems. There are many types of heart disease that could cause sudden death; chief among them is coronary heart disease or coronary artery disease. This is the end result of the accumulation of plaques that narrow the arteries supplying your heart muscle with oxygen and nutrients.

Heart disease is the leading cause of death for people in the United States. One type of heart disease is called coronary heart disease (CHD), which is caused by atherosclerosis. CHD results in narrowing of coronary arteries (through which oxygen-rich blood and nutrients are supplied to the heart). In time, the inadequate supply of oxygen-rich blood and nutrients damages the heart muscle and can lead to chest pain, heart attack, and possibly to death. If you have diabetes, high blood pressure, or elevated cholesterol, you're already at higher risk for having a heart attack, according to the National Cholesterol Education Program.

Most people with coronary heart disease show no evidence of disease for decades as the disease progresses, but there are some factors that predispose people to a greater likelihood of having the disease. For a self-managed risk assessment based on guidelines established by the National Institutes of Health's National Cholesterol Education Program (NCEP), go to http://hp2010.nhlbihin.net/atpiii/calculator.asp. Here you can calculate your risk of having a heart attack within the next ten years through your answers to seven simple questions. Another resource to assess your ten-year CHD risk is the NHLBI Framingham test, at: http://www.nhlbi.nih.gov/about/framingham/riskabs.htm. (This algorithm is based on data from a predominantly Caucasian population, without previous heart disease.) In general, the higher your score, the higher your risk for developing heart disease.

Cardiovascular Risk Score

Take note of your level of risk based on a combination of tests and the results of your physical and rank that as high, moderate, low. Please consult our list of recommendations for those with risk factors on page 231 when designing your exercise program.

Body Composition Assessment

Jen had been obese, had had gastric bypass surgery, and had lost 80 pounds. She was walking five or six times a week—about 25 miles—and had started doing marathons. Then she started lifting weights two times a week to add some resistance training to her routine to help reduce her abdominal fat and her risk for heart disease. Then, she started gaining weight. Jen got stressed and stopped lifting weights.

When she saw me next, I said, "Why did you stop?"

"Because I was gaining weight," she said.

"But how did you feel when you were putting on your clothes?" I asked.

"Actually, they were loose," she admitted. "But I was getting heavy. Since I'm always looking at my weight, the biggest stress is when I see my scale going up."

In fact, Jen was gaining muscle—lean body mass—which is good for weight loss in the long term because the more muscle you have the more calories you burn. She was building lean body mass, and lean body mass weighs more than fat, so weight gain is a necessary phase to go through. Unfortunately, by the time I saw her she had not been lifting for a while and had already lost the lean body mass she had gained through strength training and needed to start from the beginning.

—Max

That's the trouble with using weight to measure your success.

"Weighing" your progress in losing fat and gaining lean body mass by weighing yourself alone can be misleading. Your scale doesn't differentiate a pound of fat from a pound of muscle. A measure that is often used to assess your baseline before starting a diet and/or an exercise program is the Body Mass Index (BMI). BMI is *not* your body composition. Your BMI is instead the ratio of your weight with the square of your height to determine a number, which correlates to your body density.

Think of a marathoner, tall and light. He will score a low BMI. However, a short bodybuilder, with little fat but a lot of "heavy" muscles, will score a high BMI. Measuring your BMI is better than just measuring your body weight. By considering the additional factor of height, you learn more about yourself. Two hundred pounds of body weight impact a 5'2" frame differently than a 6'5" person. By using the BMI, research can also compare groups of people of different height and weight. For example, we learned that in women over age fifty a low BMI increases the risk of osteoporosis, or that a BMI above 25 goes hand in hand with increased risk for heart disease. We could not delineate those risks based simply on women of a certain weight. In athletes, BMI also tells us a lot about performance. A cyclist with a BMI of 19–20 would be a great climber but will suffer when going fast on flats with a strong headwind.

Using your height and weight, find your BMI on the following chart appropriate to your gender, and make note of it. The shaded areas indicate the healthy BMI range.

BODY MASS INDEX CHART FEMALE

Height (in.) Weight (lb.)	49	51	53	55	57	59	61	63	65	67	69	71	73	75	77	79	81	83
66	19	18	16	15	14	13	12	12	11	10	10	9	9	8	8	8	7	7
70	20	19	18	16	15	14	13	13	12	11	10	10	9	9	8	8	8	7
75	22	20	19	17	16	15	14	13	12	12	11	10	10	9	9	9	8	8
79	23	21	20	18	17	16	15	14	13	12	12	11	11	10	9	9	9	8
84	24	22	21	19	18	17	16	15	14	13	12	12	11	11	10	10	9	9
88	26	24	22	20	19	18	17	16	15	14	13	12	12	11	11	10	10	9
92	27	25	23	21	20	19	17	16	15	15	14	13	12	12	11	11	10	10
97	28	26	24	22	21	20	18	17	16	15	14	14	13	12	12	11	10	10
101	29	27	25	23	22	20	19	18	17	16	15	14	13	13	12	12	11	10
106	31	28	26	24	23	21	20	19	18	17	16	15	14	13	13	12	11	11
110	32	30	27	26	24	22	21	20	18	17	16	15	15	14	13	13	11	11
114	33	31	29	27	25	23	22	20	19	18	17	16	15	14	14	13	12	12
119	35	32	30	28	26	24	22	21	20	19	18	17	16	15	14	14	13	12
123	36	33	31	29	27	25	23	22	21	19	18	17	16	16	15	14	13	13
128	37	34	32	30	28	26	24	23	21	20	19	18	17	16	15	15	14	13
132	38	36	33	31	29	27	25	23	22	21	20	19	18	17	16	15	14	14
136	40	37	34	32	29	28	26	24	23	21	20	19	18	17	16	16	15	14
141	41	38	35	33	30	28	27	25	24	22	21	20	19	18	17	16	15	15
145	42	39	36	34	31	29	27	26	24	23	22	20	19	18	17	17	16	15
150	44	40	37	35	32	30	28	27	25	24	22	21	20	19	18	17	16	15
154	45	41	38	36	33	31	29	27	26	24	23	22	20	19	18	18	17	16
158	46	43	40	37	34	32	30	28	26	25	24	22	21	20	19	18	17	16
163	47	44	41	38	35	33	31	29	27	26	24	23	22	20	19	19	18	17
167	49	45	42	39	36	34	32	30	28	26	25	23	22	21	20	19	18	17
172	50	46	43	40	37	35	32	30	29	27	25	24	23	22	21	20	19	18
176	51	47	44	41	38	36	33	31	29	28	26	25	23	22	21	20	19	18
180	52	49	45	42	39	36	34	32	30	28	27	25	24	23	22	21	20	19
185	54	50	46	43	40	37	35	33	31	29	27	26	25	23	22	21	20	19
189	55	51	47	44	41	38	36	34	32	30	28	27	25	24	23	22	20	20
194	56	52	48	45	42	39	37	34	32	30	29	27	26	24	23	22	21	20
198	58	53	49	46	43	40	37	35	33	31	29	28	26	25	24	23	21	20
202	59	54	50	47	44	41	38	36	34	32	30	28	27	25	24	23	22	21
207	60	56	52	48	45	42	39	37	35	33	31	29	27	26	25	24	22	21
211	61	57	53	49	46	43	40	38	35	33	31	30	28	27	25	24	23	22
216	63	58	54	50	47	44	41	38	36	34	32	30	29	27	26	25	23	22
220	34	59	55	51	48	44	42	39	37	35	33	31	29	28	26	25	24	23
224	65	60	56	52	49	45	42	40	37	35	33	31	30	28	27	26	24	23
229	67	62	57	53	49	46	43	41	38	36	34	32	30	29	27	26	25	24
233	68	63	58	54	50	47	44	41	39	37	35	33	31	29	28	27	25	24
238	69	64	59	55	51	48	45	42	40	37	35	33	32	30	28	27	26	24
242	70	65	60	56	52	49	46	43	40	38	36	34	32	30	29	28	26	25
246	72	66	61	57	53	50	47	44	41	39	37	35	33	31	29	28	27	25
251	73	67	63	58	54	51	47	45	42	39	37	35	33	32	30	29	27	26
255	74	69	64	59	55	52	48	45	43	40	38	36	34	32	31	29	28	26
260	76	70	65	60	56	52	49	46	43	41	39	36	34	33	31	30	28	27
264	77	71	66	61	57	53	50	47	44	42	39	37	35	33	32	30	29	27
268	78	72	67	62	58	54	51	48	45	42	40	38	36	34	32	31	29	28
273	79	73	68	63	59	55	52	48	46	43	40	38	36	34	33	31	30	28
277	81	75	69	64	60	56	52	49	46	44	41	39	37	35	33	32	30	29
282	82	76	70	65	61	57	53	50	47	44	42	40	37	35	34	32	30	29
286	83	77	71	66	62	58	54	51	48	45	42	40	38	36	34	33	31	29
290	84	78	72	67	63	59	55	52	48	46	43	41	39	37	35	33	31	30
295	86	79	74	68	64	60	56	52	49	46	44	41	39	37	35	34	32	30
299	87	80	75	69	65	60	57	53	50	47	44	42	40	38	36	34	32	31
304	88	82	76	70	66	61	57	54	51	48	45	43	40	38	36	35	33	31
308	90	83	77	71	67	62	58	55	51	48	46	43	41	39	37	35	33	32

BODY MASS INDEX CHART MALE

Height (in.)	49	51	53	55	57	59	61	63	65	67	69	71	73	75	77	79	81	83
Weight (lb.)																		
66	19	18	16	15	14	13	12	12	11	10	10	9	9	8	8	8	7	7
70	20	19	18	16	15	14	13	13	12	11	10	10	9	9	8	8	8	7
75	22	20	19	17	16	15	14	13	12	12	11	10	10	9	9	9	8	8
79	23	21	20	18	17	16	15	14	13	12	12	11	11	10	9	9	9	8
84	24	22	21	19	18	17	16	15	14	13	12	12	11	11	10	10	9	9
88	26	24	22	20	19	18	17	16	15	14	13	12	12	11	11	10	10	9
92	27	25	23	21	20	19	17	16	15	15	14	13	12	12	11	11	10	10
97	28	26	24	22	21	20	18	17	16	15	14	14	13	12	12	11	10	10
101	29	27	25	23	22	20	19	18	17	16	15	14	13	13	12	12	11	10
106	31	28	26	24	23	21	20	19	18	17	16	15	14	13	13	12	11	11
110	32	30	27	26	24	22	21	20	18	17	16	15	15	14	13	13	11	11
114	33	31	29	27	25	23	22	20	19	18	17	16	15	14	14	13	12	12
119	35	32	30	28	26	24	22	21	20	19	18	17	16	15	14	14	13	12
123	36	33	31	29	27	25	23	22	21	19	18	17	16	16	15	14	13	13
128	37	34	32	30	28	26	24	23	21	20	19	18	17	16	15	15	14	13
132	38	36	33	31	29	27	25	23	22	21	20	19	18	17	16	15	14	14
136	40	37	34	32	29	28	26	24	23	21	20	19	18	17	16	16	15	14
141	41	38	35	33	30	28	27	25	24	22	21	20	19	18	17	16	15	15
145	42	39	36	34	31	29	27	26	24	23	22	20	19	18	17	17	16	15
150	44	40	37	35	32	30	28	27	25	24	22	21	20	19	18	17	16	15
154	45	41	38	36	33	31	29	27	26	24	23	22	20	19	18	18	17	16
158	46	43	40	37	34	32	30	28	26	25	24	22	21	20	19	18	17	16
163	47	44	41	38	35	33	31	29	27	26	24	23	22	20	19	19	18	17
167	49	45	42	39	36	34	32	30	28	26	25	23	22	21	20	19	18	17
172	50	46	43	40	37	35	32	30	29	27	25	24	23	22	21	20	19	18
176	51	47	44	41	38	36	33	31	29	28	26	25	23	22	21	20	19	18
180	52	49	45	42	39	36	34	32	30	28	27	25	24	23	22	21	20	19
185	54	50	46	43	40	37	35	33	31	29	27	26	25	23	22	21	20	19
189	55	51	47	44	41	38	36	34	32	30	28	27	25	24	23	22	20	20
194	56	52	48	45	42	39	37	34	32	30	29	27	26	24	23	22	21	20
198	58	53	49	46	43	40	37	35	33	31	29	28	26	25	24	23	21	20
202	59	54	50	47	44	41	38	36	34	32	30	28	27	25	24	23	22	21
207	60	56	52	48	45	42	39	37	35	33	31	29	27	26	25	25	22	21
211	61	57	53	49	46	43	40	38	35	33	31	30	28	27	25	24	23	22
216	63	58	54	50	47	44	41	38	36	34	32	30	29	27	26	25	23	22
220	34	59	55	51	48	44	42	39	37	35	33	31	29	28	26	25	24	23
224	65	60	56	52	49	45	42	40	37	35	33	31	30	28	27	26	24	23
229	67	62	57	53	49	46	43	41	38	36	34	32	30	29	27	26	25	24
233	68	63	58	54	50	47	44	41	39	37	35	33	31	29	28	27	25	24
238	69	64	59	55	51	48	45	42	40	37	35	33	32	30	28	27	26	24
242	70	65	60	56	52	49	46	43	40	38	36	34	32	30	29	28	26	25
246	72	66	61	57	53	50	47	44	41	39	37	35	33	31	29	28	27	25
251	73	67	63	58	54	51	47	45	42	39	37	35	33	32	30	29	27	26
255	74	69	64	59	55	52	48	45	43	40	38	36	34	32	31	29	28	26
260	76	70	65	60	56	52	49	46	43	41	39	36	34	33	31	30	28	27
264	77	71	66	61	57	53	50	47	44	42	39	37	35	33	32	30	29	27
268	78	72	67	62	58	54	51	48	45	42	40	38	36	34	32	31	29	28
273	79	73	68	63	59	55	52	48	46	43	40	38	36	34	33	31	30	28
277	81	75	69	64	60	56	52	49	46	44	41	39	37	35	33	32	30	29
282	82	76	70	65	61	57	53	50	47	44	42	40	37	35	34	32	30	29
286	83	77	71	66	62	58	54	51	48	45	42	40	38	36	34	33	31	29
290	84	78	72	67	63	59	55	52	48	46	43	41	39	37	35	33	31	30
295	86	79	74	68	64	60	56	52	49	46	44	41	39	37	35	34	32	30
299	87	80	75	69	65	60	57	53	50	47	44	42	40	38	36	34	32	31
304	88	82	76	70	66	61	57	54	51	48	45	43	40	38	36	35	33	31
308	90	83	77	71	67	62	58	55	51	48	46	43	41	39	37	35	33	32

Knowing your BMI is useful, however, BMI, like body weight alone, doesn't pinpoint the composition of your body: how much is fat or muscle. A BMI of 30 (which is in the obese range on BMI charts) can be scored by very muscular bodybuilders or a person of the same height with tremendous excess fat. For these reasons we recommend tracking your progress by assessing your body composition and your BMI rather than weight alone. Your body composition is a number that reflects your fat percentage, which is the ratio of fat to total body mass. Women typically have a much higher body fat ratio than men. The minimum percent body fat considered safe and acceptable for good health is 5 percent for males and 12 percent for females—quite a difference. The average adult body fat is closer to 12 to 18 percent for men and 20 to 24 percent for women.

This test is important because the vast majority of fitness-seekers, even those who are quite knowledgeable, have no idea about how to properly gauge their body composition (or their body fat percentage) which is so important to truly measuring fitness. This is also key to measuring your progress, which is so important to motivation. By assessing your body fat composition before beginning an exercise program and as you progress, you will see that you are losing fat and gaining lean body mass as you exercise. Too many people mistakenly gauge their fitness or progress based on their weight. We aren't going to let you make that mistake!

There are several accurate means of assessing body composition or fat percentage. Choose one of the following:

1. **Bioimpedance.** If you want to track your body fat percentage on a more finite scale, on a daily basis, there are home bathroom scales, ranging from $50 to $200, which measure your fat percentage by using a technology called bioimpedance. This technology gauges body composition by measuring electrical signals as they pass through fat and lean mass. To get the most accurate rating from such a scale, be sure to weigh yourself at the same time every day. Also if you are dehydrated, your body will offer more resistance to the current, and the machine will measure you as fatter (fat offers higher internal resistance than lean body mass). You will score leaner if you drink water beforehand. Thus, always drink eight ounces of water fifteen minutes before stepping on the scale. We will also ask that, to keep an accurate track of progress, you always test under the same circumstances, such as upon rising each morning versus testing sometimes just before bed and at other times after returning from a two-mile afternoon walk.

2. **Skin fold**. Simple and quick, this way to assess fat percentage is often offered in performance labs, gyms, and health clubs. It is not the most accurate method, and its accuracy depends on the experience of the tester and the algorithm used for the assessment. However, if you have the same person testing you over time, you will have "consistent inconsistencies," so you can easily and inexpensively monitor your changes.

3. **Hydrostatic weighing**. After taking your body weight on a scale, you are lowered into a tank until all your body parts are underwater. The underwater weight is then recorded. This procedure is repeated several times to get a precise underwater weight measure. Then your body density is calculated and, with that number, your percentage of body fat is determined. The downside of this method is the inconvenience of being submerged in water.

4. **BOD POD**. This method (which uses air displacement) is a very accurate way to measure your fat percentage and also your resting metabolic rate (how many calories your body burns in a resting condition). You can probably find a lab or medical facility that uses this technology near you. It is a little more expensive than the previous methods, but it's more precise.

5. **Dual-Energy X-Ray Absorptiometry (DEXA)**. This technology differentiates body weight into the components of lean mass, fat mass, and bone. It is based on the differential absorption by tissues of two levels of X-rays. This method is very precise and reliable. DEXA can also measure regional as well as whole body fat percentage composition. It also allows measurement of bone mineral density. DEXA is considered the gold standard, and the latest body composition research uses this method. The downside is the cost and the need to ensure you have trained staff operating the machine.

Fitness Assessments

To determine your exercise prescription (intensity, volume, and frequency), we offer simple tests in each of four categories: flexibility, muscular strength, aerobic fitness, and balance and coordination. These tests will help you assess your starting point and your strengths and weaknesses. You can either do the self-managed tests we detail here, or go to a physiology lab or a certified trainer to have them performed. We start with cardiovascular fitness.

If you scored a moderate to high level of risk for heart attack when taking the Cardiovascular Risk Assessment, consult with your physician and have a supervised stress test performed before you take these tests.

Warning:

If at any point during exercise you experience light-headedness, chest pain, or difficulty breathing:

■ Don't panic.
■ Stop exercising.
■ Sit or lie down.
■ Ask for help.

Keep your legs slightly elevated, if possible. Even if the sensation passes, seek medical attention.

Cardiovascular Fitness

Your cardiovascular fitness score tells you how efficient your oxygen-carrying system is in delivering oxygen to your working muscles. It depends on the combined performance of your heart, lungs, and blood. There are many ways to assess your cardiovascular fitness. You can have your maximal oxygen uptake (VO2max) measured at a performance lab, or you can use these simple tests to estimate it.

One of the most popular cardiovascular assessments is the classic walking test. No matter your fitness level, you can perform it because this is not a test to exhaust yourself, which is not a good idea (or an attractive proposition) if you have not been exercising regularly. You take this test walking at a pace that is comfortable for you.

Choose a location for your test. Any of the following will work:

■ Out-of-doors on a *flat* stretch of road or trail that has mile markers or that you measure with your car's odometer, or using a pedometer

- On a treadmill
- In a mall using a pedometer
- At the local high school or college track (four laps equal one mile)

Preparation

- Get cleared by your physician for walking a mile if you have a known medical condition or a high-risk score.
- Wear good walking shoes and comfortable clothing.
- Drink water before, but avoid taking the test right after a meal.
- Avoid coffee or any caffeinated drinks. These can lower your score by raising your heart rate.
- Wear a watch that measures time in seconds.
- Warm up with easy walking for a few minutes.
- Practice taking your pulse on your wrist or at one side of your windpipe, using two fingertips. (Never simultaneously press both sides of your neck when you take your pulse; this can cause a drop in heart rate and blood pressure in some people.) When you feel your pulse, look at your watch and count the number of beats you feel in ten seconds. Multiply this number by six. This is your heart rate. Twenty beats, for example, multiplied by six means your heart rate is 120 beats per minute. You can also use a heart rate monitor, an electronic device that measures your heart rate.

Instructions

- Note your start time.
- Now walk your mile at a comfortable pace.
- Note your ending time.
- Immediately upon finishing, take your pulse.

You should have two numbers now:

- The time it took you to walk the mile
- Your ending heart rate

No matter the intensity at which you did the test, the combination of these two numbers will reveal your aerobic capacity. For example, if you are very fit but you don't want to push yourself you might walk the mile in twenty minutes, but your pulse might be only 100, revealing that this was easy for you. If you are someone who gives everything to walk the mile—you work hard and you end up walking the mile in fourteen minutes, your pulse at the end might be 170, revealing the level of effort this required of you.

On the following charts, find your cardiovascular fitness level using your age and the two numbers you recorded.

Your heart rate and pace will improve as you become more fit. Be aware that this measurement of aerobic fitness is somewhat imprecise because it relies on using a standardized range for heart rate as the indicator of exercise intensity, though heart rate is a parameter that differs greatly from person to person. However, this test is useful for several reasons:

- You can do it yourself.
- It provides a good, general sense of your fitness level.
- It's effective as a means of monitoring your progress over time.

Due to its imprecision, this test cannot be used for comparing yourself to someone else, however. Likewise it's not useful for comparing your results with those you get from lab tests, say, six months from now. However, this measurement of cardiovascular fitness remains constant for the same person over time—it's "consistently inconsistent," so you can retest yourself using the same test and accurately gauge your progress.

VO2max Assessment

If you want to get more sophisticated and estimate your VO2max using this walking test, there is an easy way to do it. We advise you do a test of this kind at least every year.

Among elite athletes, VO2max is considered one measure of the aerobic or endurance athletic potential; you do not know your full potential until you know your VO2max. VO2max is one of the best indicators of your aerobic fitness. Knowing your VO2max is not entirely necessary for starting an exercise program, but as you get acquainted with your body through fitness, you may become quite infatuated and find yourself wanting to know *every*thing.

There are two formulas to assess your VO2max. You can just look at the absolute amount of oxygen your body can use in a unit of time, say, in liters per minute. However, this approach gives a bonus to people of

MEN				
AGE	HEART RATE	1–2 STARS	3 STARS	4–5 STARS
20–29	110	>19:36	17:06–19:36	<17.06
	120	>19:10	16:36–19:10	<16.36
	130	>18:35	16:06–18:35	<16:06
	140	>18:06	15:36–18:06	<15:36
	150	>17:36	15:10–17:36	<15:10
	160	>17:09	14:42–17:09	<14:42
	170	>16:39	14:12–16:39	<14:12
30–39	110	>18:21	15:54–18:21	<15:54
	120	>17:52	15:24–17:52	<15:24
	130	>17:22	14:54–17:22	<14:54
	140	>16:54	14:30–16:54	<14:30
	150	>16:26	14:00–16:26	<14:00
	160	>15:58	13:30–15:58	<13:30
	170	>15:28	13:01–15:28	<13:01

40–49	110	>18:05	15:38–18:05	<15:38
	120	>17:36	15:09–17:36	<15:09
	130	:07	14:41–17:07	<14:41
	140	>16:38	14:12–16:38	<14:12
	150	>16:09	13:42–16:09	<13:42
	160	>15:42	13:15–15:42	<13:15
50–59	110	>17:49	15:22–17:49	<15:22
	120	>17:20	14:53–17:20	<14:53
	130	>16:51	14:24–16:51	<14:24
	140	>16:22	13:51–16:22	<13:51
	150	>15:53	13:26–15:53	<13:26
	160	>15:26	12:59–15:26	<12:59
	170	>14:56	12:30–14:56	<12:30
60+	110	>17:55	15:33–17:55	<15:33
	120	>17:24	15:04–17:24	<15:04
	130	>16:57	14:36–16:57	<14:36
	140	>16:28	14:07–16:28	<14:07
	150	>15:59	13:39–15:59	<13:39
	160	>15:30	13:10–15:30	<13:10
	170	>15:04	12:42–15:04	<12:42

WOMEN				
AGE	HEART RATE	1–2 STARS	3 STARS	4–5 STARS
20–29	110	> 20:57	19:08–20:57	< 19:08
	120	> 20:27	18:38–20:27	< 18:38
	130	> 20:00	18:12–20:00	< 18:12
	140	> 19:30	17:42–19:30	< 17:42
	150	> 19:00	17:12–19:00	< 17:12
	160	> 18:30	16:42–18:30	< 16:42
	170	> 18:00	16:12–18:00	< 16:12
30–39	110	> 19:46	17:52–19:40	< 17:52
	120	> 19:18	17:24–19:18	< 17:24
	130	> 18:48	16:54–18:48	< 16:54
	140	> 18:18	16:24–18:18	< 16:24
	150	> 17:48	15:54–17:48	< 15:54
	160	> 17:18	15:24–17:18	< 15:24
	170	> 15:54	14:55–16:64	< 14:55

40–49	110	> 19:15	17:20–19:15	< 17:20
	120	> 18:45	16:50–18:45	< 16:50
	130	> 18:18	16:24–18:18	< 16:24
	140	> 17:48	15:54–17:48	< 15:54
	150	> 17:18	15:24–17:18	< 15:24
	160	> 16:48	14:54–16:48	< 14:54
	170	> 16:18	14:25–16:18	< 14:25
50–59	110	> 18:40	17:04–18:40	< 17:04
	120	> 18:12	16:36–18:12	< 16:36
	130	> 17:42	16:06–17:42	< 16:06
	140	> 17:18	15:36–17:18	< 15:36
	150	> 16:48	15:06–16:48	< 15:06
	160	> 16:18	14:36–16:18	< 14:36
	170	> 15:48	14:06–15:48	< 14:06
60+	110	> 18:00	16:36–18:00	< 16:36
	120	> 17:30	16:06–17:30	< 16:06
	130	> 17:01	15:37–17:01	< 15:37
	140	> 16:31	15:09–16:31	< 15:09
	150	> 16:02	14:39–16:02	< 14:39
	160	> 15:32	14:12–15:32	< 14:12
	170	> 15:04	13:42–15:04	< 13:42

bigger size, even if their "big engine" is not quite big enough to propel their heavy body. For this reason, we prefer to correct that VO2 number for your body weight. We will express your score as milliliters of oxygen per kilogram of body weight you use every minute (mlO2/kg/min). You may simply substitute pounds for kilos and the result is almost exactly the same, because weight in the formula is multiplied by such a tiny number. However, if you want to be extremely precise you can multiply your weight in pounds by 0.45359237 to arrive at your weight in kilograms. For your gender, enter 1 if you're male and 0 if you're female.

From the walking test, use the following formula to arrive at your estimated VO2max:

$$VO2max = 132.853 - (0.0769 \times \text{Weight in pounds or kilos}) - (0.3877 \times \text{Age}) + (6.31 \times \text{Gender}) - (3.2649 \times \text{Time}) - (0.1565 \times \text{Heart rate})$$

This calculation is a good option for people who don't have access to a lab; however, be aware that this formula will yield your *estimated* VO2max. It is arrived at from measuring other parameters, namely your heart rate, pace, and age; it's not your direct VO2max measurement. But the parameters correlate well enough with your actual VO2max that you can use it repeatedly to track your improvement over time. In other words, it may overestimate your VO2max or underestimate it, but the error will be consistent. Like the heart rate test, you cannot use this estimation of VO2max to compare one person to another.

Lab VO2max Assessment

Lab tests are the gold standard for assessing VO2max. With a lab test, you get a quite precise, direct measurement. If you have never had your VO2max measured, it's worth doing. If you already have been tested, it's worthwhile to have your VO2max measured annually. The cost for a supervised VO2max test is relatively low. In most cases it's about the cost of a pair of running shoes. If you have symptoms such as shortness of breath during exercise or your physician has recommended you have a medical assessment in a lab, you can ask for this test as part of your medical assessment, and your insurance will pay for it in most cases.

If you don't feel comfortable going to a lab now because you're very out of shape, we assure you that the best time to get tested *is* when you're out of shape because you will get your best baseline measurements before you start to exercise. Lots of people call us who would like to come for testing and they say, "I want to know my VO2max, but I'm out of shape.

How many weeks should I train before you can give me an accurate test?"

And I say, "No, you should come right now. I want to see where you are now. Then you can come back in three or six months and I can tell you how much you have improved with training. I want to see if the training program is making a difference or if I need to figure out a different way to train you because you don't respond to the traditional approach."

There are lots of ways labs can measure VO2max. To get the most out of your assessment you'll want to ask for a VO2max test with an assessment of your ventilatory threshold. Your ventilatory threshold is the point where you start breathing significantly harder in an attempt to deliver to your muscles the amount of oxygen they require for that level of effort.

If you think of your VO2max as the size of your engine, your ventilatory threshold is the percentage of that engine you can use on a long drive (for example, some cars have a turbo that kicks in though the engine size remains the same). Knowing your ventilatory threshold pinpoints your training zones.

Many people are intimidated about selecting the right lab for this kind of testing. To get what you need out of your lab test, be sure that the lab meets the following criteria.

The Right Lab for the Right Test

- Your tests should be supervised by a doctor, an exercise physiologist, a registered nurse, or an ECG tech. This is a *must* if you have a known heart disease, ten years of inactivity behind you, you're overweight, or you have high blood pressure, diabetes, or elevated cholesterol.
- The lab should be in a health club with staff trained to respond to cardiac events, or in a medical setting, such as a clinic or a hospital.
- You will find the most accurate equipment for measuring VO2max at a human performance lab at a local college or university, or at a sports performance or medical center with a good reputation for working with athletes.

At the lab ask for:

- A VO2max test with an assessment of your ventilatory threshold.
- Your individualized training zones, and how to use them (for example, if your goal is to lose weight, ask for the intensity or heart rate range

where you are burning more calories from fat, based on your metabolic response).

■ Your blood pressure during rest and exercise.

■ An ongoing ECG during the test if you are at high risk for heart disease.

VO2max Score

Once you have arrived at your VO2max estimate based on your numbers from the aerobic assessment (walking test) or have received your results from your lab tests, you will want to know where you stand and your potential for improvement.

If your VO2max is:

Under 20 = You are definitely unfit. You may want to rule out a medical condition that maybe limiting you aerobically, such as heart or lung disease. It is possible that you are overweight (a large weight drops the VO2-to-weight ratio number).

25 to 35 = You are sedentary to average in aerobic fitness.

35 to 44 = You have above average aerobic fitness, that of someone who dedicates 3–5 hours a week to aerobic activity.

45 to 49 = You are definitely fit.

50 to 60 = You might be a competitive endurance athlete, a potential marathoner.

60 to 70 = You might be a national-level athlete.

70 to 80 = You might be an international-level athlete, a Tour de France rider.

Above 80 = You are one of the few, matching the scores of the top endurance athletes in the world.

Above 90 = Those who score in the 90s are genetically gifted and highly trained top athletes in cross-country skiing, cycling, or mid- to long-distance running—that's where we see the highest scores.

Eric's was 85 when he was skating; now he's probably in the upper 50s, low 60s. Max's is between 45 and 50.

Now compare your VO2max to the chart here to get a sense of your overall aerobic fitness level according to your age, from 1 to 5 stars.

MEN

Age	*	**	***	****	*****
20-29	below 37.8	38.9 to 43.1	44.1 to 51.1	51.8 to 56	over 57.1
30-39	below 34	35.4 to 38.9	39.9 to 46.9	48 to 51.1	over 51.8
40-49	below 30.1	30.8 to 35	36.1 to 43.1	44.1 to 46.9	over 48
50-59	below 24.9	25.9 to 30.8	31.9 to 38.9	39.9 to 43.1	over 44.1
60-69	below 21	22.1 to 25.9	27 to 35	36.1 to 38.9	over 39.9

WOMEN

Age	*	**	***	****	*****
20-29	below 28	29 to 34	35 to 43	44.1 to 48	30-39
30-39	below 27	28 to 32.9	34 to 41	42 to 46.9	over 48
40-49	below 24.9	25.9 to 30.8	31.9 to 39.9	41 to 44.8	over 45.9
50-59	below 21	22.1 to 27	28 to 36.1	37.1 to 41	over 42
60-69	below 16.8	17.9 to 22.1	23.1 to 30.8	31.9 to 36.1	over 37.1

Best Activity Choices for High VO2max

A high VO2max will serve you well in all activities in which you have to sustain an effort for more than four or five minutes at high intensity and that involve the use of a high percentage of your muscle mass. If you have a high VO2max, some of the activities you will excel in include cross-country skiing, mid- and long-distance running, rowing, swimming, cycling, and skating (especially longer-distance speed skating).

Best Activity Choices for Mid-Range VO2max

People with an intermediate VO2max level can do well at team sports. You don't need a high VO2max to play baseball, for example, or soccer, basketball, or rugby. Though some of these sports require that you will have to run for several minutes at a time, your skill level is key, but you only need to have a decent VO2max. A national-level soccer player has a VO2max in the 55–65 range, a great score but not as high as that of a Tour de France cyclist.

However, if you want to improve your VO2max, pick one of those activities we mentioned, such as cycling, running, swimming, or rowing.

Best Activity Choices for Low VO2max

People with a low VO2max can do well in any activity that requires efforts that last fewer than two or three minutes. These don't require a high VO2max. If you have a low VO2max, you can still be very fast and very strong, and could do well as a sprinter in events such as the 100-meter dash or in weight lifting. A high VO2max is not required in any sport where you need tremendous muscle strength or power for a short time. Football and volleyball players, baseball players and sprinters may also have low VO2max because their efforts are short and they have time to recover in between. These sports instead require more skill than endurance.

Importance of Improving Your VO2max

No matter which activities you choose, it's always beneficial to improve your VO2max. Because your VO2max goes along with your body's ability to recover, training your VO2max is never a bad thing. Say you are a sprinter who does the 100-meter dash. When training you will have to run plenty of sprints: 60 meters, 80 meters, 100 meters, 200 meters. You will want to work hard, and your ability to recover from each of those bursts of anaerobic activity will be determined by your aerobic fitness. On race day, you probably don't need a high VO2max because you'll run only 100 or 200 meters, and then have hours to rest before your next race. But in order to be able to run your fastest 100-meter race, you have to be able to train hard and that requires good recovery. The training load will be easier on you if you have a better

VO2max. For this reason, we instruct you to work on establishing a good aerobic base and improving your VO2max, no matter the activity you choose.

How to Improve Your VO2max

You can improve your VO2max 15 to 25 percent by stressing your oxygen-carrying system three to six times a week. The range of your potential VO2max is primarily genetically determined, but where it falls within that spectrum is a matter of your level of aerobic fitness. If you are completely out of shape and sitting at the bottom of your range, you could improve your VO2max 20 to 30 percent, sometimes more if you also lose a good deal of weight. That means that if you were born with a potential for a VO2max of 60–65, you can get to 75–80 with good training. If you were born with 35 you could perhaps achieve 45 or 50 with training, 55 if you also lose weight. That's an astonishing improvement, yet quite attainable.

To see that kind of improvement, you need to be serious about your fitness and you need to give yourself at least six months. You will likely see substantial improvement in the first three months, but to measure significant improvement requires closer to six months, during which you have to be consistent in your training. As touched on above, losing weight also spells substantial gains. We have clients who are carrying 250 to 300 pounds, and when they drop 80 pounds, their VO2max goes up more than 30 percent, not simply because their oxygen uptake increases significantly but because they drop weight, which changes the number against which oxygen consumption is compared.

If you are already on a training schedule, competing locally in cycling, say, or soccer, or in running, you are likely at the top end of your genetic range. It's important to understand the firm genetic limits of your VO2max. As we detailed earlier, many people fall prey to the notion that if they haven't done well in certain activities it's only because they didn't push themselves hard enough. But there's no reason to be too hard on yourself; your genes set the limit on this. It's better to know and choose activities better suited to your strengths. In some countries, they measure VO2max and other parameters on highly competitive young athletes from the start in order to steer them toward sports that suit them best. It's not a bad strategy and it certainly guarantees greater success.

You cannot change your genes for now, though that may be possible down the road with progress in genetic manipulation. In the meantime, the increases in VO2max you are likely to see are in the 5 to 15 percent range, if you follow a program to do so.

With those caveats in mind, you can improve your VO2max—to the degree possible—by doing the following:

- Be physically active three to six times a week.
- Pick one of many aerobic activities (so-called because they rely on oxygen availability): running, swimming, cycling, rowing, X-C skiing, skating. These aerobic activities are at the top of the list, but intermittent activities, such as soccer, lacrosse, and rugby, are great, too.
- Keep the intensity at a level hard enough to stress your oxygen delivery system but without exhausting you too quickly. A good way to pace yourself is to use your rate of perceived exertion.

Rate of Perceived Exertion

Scientists have created a scale that defines the levels of effort you feel when exercising. It's called the rate of perceived exertion (RPE). This is another tool you'll use on your road to fitness and it's easy to apply on a daily basis.

Each step on the rate of perceived exertion scale describes a feeling and correlates it with how much work your body is doing. When you perceive your level of exertion is weak, that's a 2 on the scale; when you feel it's strong—that's 5; maximum effort—10. It's important to notice how your body feels at different levels of exertion so that you can use those feelings to place your workouts at the intensity—or level of exertion—that is prescribed for you in your program.

There are several scales of perceived exertion. We use the scientifically validated Borg scale, which looks like this:

Rating	Description
0	Nothing at all
0.5	Very, very weak
1	Very weak
2	Weak
3	Moderate
4	Somewhat strong

5 Strong
6 Between strong and very strong
7 Very strong
8 Between very strong and very, very
      strong
9 Very, very strong
10 Maximal

There is another Borg scale that rates effort between 4 and 20, but we have better results with the 0–10 version.

To get accustomed to using the RPE, try it out first under circumstances where you can pay close attention to your body's signals.

- Choose a physical activity that's comfortable for you: walking, riding a bike, or walking on a treadmill.
- Start at an easy pace.
- Slowly increase the pace until you feel you are working at an intensity that is weak or easy, that you don't have to exert much of an effort to continue. This point marks your RPE Level 2.
- Now go a little faster, until you start feeling the effort is moderate. This is Level 3 out of 10 for you on the RPE chart.
- Next, increase to an intensity that you feel is strong. This is Level 5 out of 10 on the RPE chart.
- Now increase your workout intensity to a pace that is very strong or between 6 and 7 out of 10 on the RPE chart, or "very strong" effort.

At the beginning, you may want to carry a copy of the RPE with you when you work out to ensure you exercise at the right level. The RPE is very easy to use when you want to gauge your effort. And despite its simplicity the RPE is also very accurate. When we test people in our lab using the RPE while simultaneously testing VO2max or blood lactate levels, we find that a person's rate of perceived exertion correlates closely with the person's metabolic response in 90 percent of cases. In other words, your body is good at telling you precisely how hard it's working on a chemical and metabolic level. Many people use a heart rate monitor, which is great when you know your correct training zones (not the ones based on your age) for that specific training modality (your correct heart rate zones when running are different from the ones you should use on your bike or when cross-country skiing). So, based on its accuracy and our experience, we tend to favor the use of the RPE as a way of assessing and monitoring exercise intensity—for the 90 percent of people for which it works.

For the remaining 10 percent of people, the RPE doesn't work well. The people for whom the RPE is ill suited are those who, during incremental tests in the lab, perceive their exertion as "2," then "2," then "2," then suddenly "10!" Or they might perceive the increases in their body's effort at the beginning but then jump from 3, say, all the way to 10.

If you want a precise RPE measurement, it's worth getting measured in a good lab, with expert supervision, so someone can simultaneously monitor your heart rate, blood lactate concentration, oxygen uptake, *and* RPE. From the analysis of these numbers, the lab can then also assess your individualized training zones.

Using the RPE to Determine Training Zones

You can now get a little more sophisticated and divide the RPE into training zones by correlating your heart rate with your RPE chart. If you don't wish to do this, you can also determine your zones based on the RPE chart alone (see below).

You can take your pulse or use a heart rate monitor. (We recommend using a heart rate monitor to keep track of your heart rate for this test.)

Being able to identify your training zones using the RPE is very handy because you will soon be designing your exercise program with exercise on different days and weeks prescribed in varying training zones. Performing your aerobic workouts within the right training zone is yet another tool to making the most of your time and effort, by ensuring that you're exercising the right system in the right sequence.

You establish your training zones in much the same manner as you used the RPE the first time:

- Choose a physical activity that's comfortable for you: walking, riding a bike, or walking on a treadmill.
- Start at an easy pace.
- Slowly increase the pace until you feel you are working at an intensity that is weak or easy, that you don't have to put out much of an effort to

maintain. This point marks your RPE Level 2. Hold this effort for two to three minutes and record your heart rate (HR). (If you are using a treadmill, you may want to take note of the speed in order to monitor improvement over time. As you progress with training, you should find that your speed is higher for the same RPE level.)

■ Now go a little faster, until you start feeling the effort is moderate. This is Level 3 out of 10 for you on the RPE chart. Hold this intensity for 2 to 3 minutes, and then record your HR again (and the speed if you are using a treadmill).

■ Next, increase to an intensity that you feel is strong. This is Level 5. Maintain this for 2 to 3 minutes, then take and record your heart rate (and speed).

■ Now increase your workout intensity to a pace that is very strong or between 6 and 7 out of 10 on the RPE chart, or "very strong" effort. Maintain this for three minutes, and then measure your heart rate (and speed if applicable).

Your Training Zones Based on Your Heart Rate

Following this test you should have four heart rate numbers. Say that you recorded 118, 136, 148, and 156.

Your heart rate (HR) training zones are:

Zone 1 = below 118
Zone 2 = 118–136
Zone 3 = 136–148
Zone 4 = 148–156
Zone 5 = above 156

Your Training Zones Based on Treadmill Speed Values

You may also have four treadmill speed numbers, say (in miles/hour) 5.5, 6.2, 7.0, and 7.6.

Your speed training zones are:

Zone 1 = slower than 5.5 mph
Zone 2 = 5.5–6.2 mph
Zone 3 = 6.2–7.0 mph

Zone 4 = 7.0–7.6 mph
Zone 5 = faster than 7.6 mph

Your Training Zones Based Just on RPE

If you didn't correlate the effort intensity with any heart rate or speed, just use the RPE numbers:

RPE below 2 = Zone 1
Zone 1 is termed easy aerobic. This is the way you want to feel when you are warming up or cooling down.

RPE of 2–3 = Zone 2
Exercise in Zone 2 builds what we call an aerobic base; it's also called extensive aerobic. Zone 2 is perfect for a long, easy workout. It is also the zone best for beginners and for people beginning training after a long period of inactivity. It exerts mild stress on the cardiovascular system during workouts of thirty minutes to an hour. Exercise in Zone 2 burns calories primarily from energy we have stored as fat, the highest percentage of any of the zones.

RPE of 3–5 = Zone 3
Zone 3 is hailed as the aerobic capacity zone; it's also called intensive aerobic, or the cardio-fitness zone. That is the level you'd maintain when competing in the Ironman or your first few marathons. It is also the zone you'll reach into when you first begin interval training, starting with 3 to 5 minutes in this zone, with a 3- to 5-minute rest in Zone 2 between intervals. As you progress in your efforts, you will eventually spend 30 minutes to an hour in Zone 3 as you get in more advanced condition. Zone 3 exerts a significant training effect on your cardiovascular system and on your muscles by building muscular enzymes. You also burn a good deal of calories when you are in Zone 3, and a good number of those calories are coming from fat (though as a percentage, Zone 2 burns a higher ratio of fat but fewer total calories).

Zone 3 is where you really stress your cardiovascular system in training for long efforts. To improve, you need to increase either volume or intensity. Often your time may be limited by other commitments. When your brief intervals in Zone 3 get easy, you can increase your intensity since you may not be able to increase the total time you are working out. RPE 3–5 is the feeling you want to strive to maintain the majority of the time during your workouts.

RPE of 5–7 = Zone 4

This is the aerobic-anaerobic transition zone, where both aerobic and anaerobic pathways are contributing to energy production. Part of this energy is produced without oxygen utilization. At this intensity, lactate production and reutilization rates are at a breaking point. Often this zone is referred to as the "anaerobic threshold." This is the zone you would use when competing; it is the pace you'd use in a 10k run or a half marathon. In this zone you breathe very fast and deeply; you experience some discomfort if not pain. That's because the increase of hydrogen ions causes muscle acidity and stimulates your respiratory center to breathe faster and deeper. Indeed, you get rid of the hydrogen ions by exhaling more carbon dioxide.

This zone is where top athletes spend the lion's share of their time. You want to target this feeling and work out at this intensity if you want to become competitive and seek improvement at that high level. But before you do that, you want to be able to do more work in Zone 3 in order to prepare your body to better tolerate work in Zone 4.

RPE of 8–10 = Zone 5

Called the Red Zone, "the gasping zone" or your "turbo engine," this is the zone of elite athletes. If you compete in certain sports, you are definitely spending time in Zone 5 during your races, so it makes sense to gradually get used to this level of effort during your training. However, if your goal is to improve your aerobic fitness and your overall health, you don't need to plan specific time in Zone 5. Maximum-intensity efforts of this kind could in fact have a negative impact if you have a medical condition or a predisposition to musculoskeletal injury. For this reason we also avoid the alternative way of establishing training zones: using a person's maximum heart rate.

Why Not Use Maximum Heart Rate?

Traditionally, doctors have dished out exercise using training zones based on maximum heart rates and averages. They test a patient by telling her to work up to her maximum heart rate (Zone 5), then record her heart rate (and, all too often, clean up her vomit). After this unpleasant experience, she's told to figure out her training zones by multiplying her maximum heart rate by a percentage based on what works for most people. For example, if she wants to work out in Zone 3, they tell her to just multiply her maximum heart rate by 70 to 80 percent, assuming all people are feeling the same (and their bodies are doing the same work) at 70 to 80 percent of their maximum.

This method has its obvious and not-so-obvious drawbacks. As we've mentioned, being pushed to the maximum is not comfortable for most people. In addition, any assumption of targeting a zone or intensity based on multiplying the maximum downward is based on averages, and is not specific to the individual athlete. A marathon runner, for example, can stay at 90 percent of her maximum with relatively little effort, whereas a sprinter will feel fatigue at 75 percent of his maximum.

Many people target their ideal training zones using heart rate (HR) monitors. This can be very helpful in measuring the intensity of exercise, since your HR during effort increases regularly with the increase of the amount of oxygen that your muscles require. In other words, a heart rate monitor accurately measures how fast your aerobic engine is working. The problem is assessing the heart rate ranges that are appropriate for you. As we said, in general, most people measure training zones by starting from their maximum HR (HRM), either directly measured, or estimated by a formula where a person subtracts their age from 220 and—voilà!—that's their maximum heart rate. Then, from that HRM, they establish the different zones by multiplying it by percentages, as above.

This formula is convenient and it avoids the discomfort and danger of taking your body to maximum intensity. However, everyone has a different heart rate response to exercise. Medically speaking, the 220-age formula has a standard deviation of 12 beats/min (bpm). That means that over 60 percent of the people in the same age group have an HRM within 24 bpm of one another, and 95 percent of them are within 48 bpm. That means that over half of the forty-five-year-olds, for example, will actually have a maximum heart rate that is anywhere from 163 to 187, but they will all base their training on a maximum heart rate of 175. And almost *all* of these forty-five-year-olds will actually have heart rates of 151–199, but, again, they will all be doggedly training in zones based on an HRM of 175. This tells you that the mean value of the HRM for all the subjects of the same age is not precise enough to be used for individualized training intensity assessment.

Our approach using the RPE might seem to be more complicated at a glance, but even in our lab after a long time working with patients of different training backgrounds we realized that the RPE scale is more user-friendly and reliable than assessing their training zones via their maximum heart rate. And there is less risk and less discomfort involved. When you assess your zones starting at the lowest intensity and working your way up, you don't ever have to be stressed to the maximum. Once you get to RPE 8–9, you've already established your zones, so you don't need to ever go to RPE 10. However, a physiological test performed in the lab is the gold standard for getting a more accurate reading of your own response to exercise.

When you use the RPE you also remove the willingness-to-suffer variable. When a doctor asks a patient to work up to their maximum intensity to record their heart rate, how hard the patient works is very much dependent on how motivated they are to push themselves on a given day. Your main objective here is measuring your metabolic response, not your willingness to suffer when you do a test.

For this same reason, the RPE is also ideal for measuring your progress.

Using the RPE for Measuring Progress

People who assess their progress often measure their improvement based on their time doing maximum performance, also called their "personal best." Measuring your improvement based on your best effort has its pluses, but it's not ideal for one key reason: Your score at the end of your maximum performance conveys the level of your current physical ability, yes, but—as we mentioned above—whenever you measure your progress by, say, running your best mile, your time will vary greatly, depending on how much you want to push yourself that day. You may be very excited, very positive, not at all fatigued, and see a very good outcome because that number is also very much a product of your current state of mind. Even if you have not improved your physical condition—or have even lost ability—you might score higher than the last time you tested yourself because you are mentally able to push yourself harder that day. You might improve your performance by three seconds over your last assessment. But is that a measure of your body's improvements?

Quite the opposite is true when you feel a little depressed or when you've had a bad day. Physically, you may have progressed significantly, but due to fatigue, depression, or a stressful day, in a test of your maximum performance you may score lower than your last assessment. Thus, every time you measure improvement by measuring a *maximum* performance, you are measuring the result of your brain + your body, and you can never be certain that the outcome of a test of your personal best is the result of your current physical status. In addition to the mental factors that impact maximum performance, there are other possible mitigating factors. Has your form improved? Or has your aerobic engine gotten harder? Or were you simply pushing yourself harder?

However, if you measure your progress by measuring your *sub*maximal effort, using the RPE, you measure only your body's response—your engine. So we prefer to measure submaximal effort at three different levels: very weak, moderate, and very strong but not maximum.

We recommend that you test your progress every six weeks using submaximal effort. Measure your time, power, or speed at three different RPE intensities: at a very weak pace, at a moderate pace, and at a very strong but not maximum pace. On a graph, put your RPE on the x-axis, and your speed (running, walking, swimming) or power (cycling, rowing) on the y-axis. Over time, as you improve, the line connecting these points should shift to the left. That means that for the same perceived effort, your performance (measured as speed or power) is higher. The steeper the line, the more you have improved!

Aerobic fitness level based on your score to the walking/VO2max tests:

If you scored:

1 star: It's probably no surprise to you that you are in poor aerobic condition. You need to be serious about getting exercise because the health risks to people with your level of aerobic fitness are numerous and sobering. You also need to approach fitness carefully. Your score could also be related to the fact that you don't exercise regularly. But if this score is a surprise, you may have a medical condition. You should consult with your physician or have your cardiac fitness measured through a direct VO2max or cardiopulmonary stress test. The good news is that you have the most potential for improvement.

2 stars: You have lower-than-average aerobic fitness. It could be related to the fact that you are overweight or you don't exercise regularly. If you think you are more active than this score reflects, it could be related to a medical condition. You should consult with your physician or have your

aerobic fitness measured through an actual V02max or cardiopulmonary stress test.

3 stars: You have average aerobic fitness. It's time to get better.

4 stars: You're above average. You're just below the highest level. With some more effort you may be able to reach the top.

5 stars: Good job. You're either doing a good job training or you have great potential.

Basic instructions for all levels:

> If at any point during exercise you experience light-headedness, chest pain, or difficulty breathing, don't panic, stop exercising, lie down, and ask for help. Keep your legs slightly elevated. Even if it passes, seek medical attention.

To see the biggest gains, on your calendar space your aerobic workouts as follows:

- Alternate the hard aerobic and light aerobic days.
- Slot your hardest aerobic session on the day before your complete rest day, and work strength and flexibility the day after it.
- Schedule your light aerobic sessions on the same day as flexibility training or the same day as muscular strengthening sessions that work another group of muscles (for example, schedule a brisk walk on the same day you do your upper-body strengthening).

IF YOU SCORED 1 STAR:

You are very likely a beginner to exercise and fitness. First and foremost, you need to spend time with a doctor to be sure that there is not a medical problem that is causing your lack of aerobic fitness (such as a heart condition, anemia, or asthma) or that needs to be treated before you can pursue fitness safely. If you have experienced any kind of limitation when you exercise: shortness of breath, chest pressure or light-headedness, you must be cleared by a physician before continuing.

If your doctor gives you the green light to begin an exercise program, you need to choose an aerobic activity that is easy. Walking and swimming are good options. If you have musculoskeletal problems, such as bad knees, you may want to consider bicycle riding on flat roads, using an elliptical trainer if you have access to a gym, or swimming and aquaerobics if you have access to a pool. In general, take every opportunity to move. Take the dog for a walk, mow the lawn, do some gardening.

As you work your way steadily through your exercise program, you must give your body time to adapt to the increasing effort.

Remember, you have the greatest potential to improve.

Weeks 1–3

You will want to calendar:

- A walk, swim, or ride every second day or 3–4 days a week.
- Warm-up for 10 minutes each day in Zone 1.
- Workout for 15 to 20 minutes in Zone 2.
- Never go above Zone 2.

To improve, gradually increase your intensity (speed) or distance in small increments, say 10 percent every week. But remember that the goal is not how long or how hard you go, it's that you are getting out and moving, and every time you move you do some good. You improve your cardiovascular and muscular fitness and increase your bone density.

Weeks 4–5

- Add one aerobic workout, so you are now doing 4–5.
- Warm up each day for 10 minutes in Zone 1.
- Increase one of the 4 to 5 workouts to 30 minutes in Zone 2.
- To improve your aerobic capacity, do one of the shorter, 20-minute days, at a higher intensity, alternating 3 minutes in Zone 3 with 3 minutes in Zone 2.

Week 6

- Train every second day, for a total of 3 to 4 times per week.
- Always warm up for 10 minutes in Zone 1.
- Increase one of the workouts to 40 minutes in Zone 2.
- The other days, work out for 30 minutes, alternating 4 minutes in Zone 3 with 2 minutes in Zone 2.

Weeks 7–9

- Do 5 workouts.
- Always warm up for 10 minutes in Zone 1.
- Do two 30-minute workouts, alternating 4 minutes in Zone 3 with 2 minutes in Zone 2.
- Do two 45-minute workouts in Zone 2.
- Do one workout with 3 efforts alternating 3 minutes in Zone 4, separated by 4-minute recoveries in Zone 2.

Week 10

- Train every second day, for a total of 3 to 4 times (this is a recovery week).
- Always warm up for 10 minutes in Zone 1.
- Do two 40-minute workouts in Zone 2.
- Do one 30-minute workout, alternating 4 minutes in Zone 3 with 2 minutes in Zone 2.
- Do one workout alternating 3 efforts of 4 minutes each in Zone 4 with 4-minute recoveries in Zone 2.

Weeks 11–12

- Add one aerobic workout, so you are now back to doing 4 to 5 again.
- Warm up each day for 10 minutes in Zone 1.
- Do two 45-minute workouts in Zone 2, with the last 5 minutes in Zone 3.
- Do two 30-minute workouts, alternating 6 minutes in Zone 3 with 2 minutes in Zone 2.
- Do one workout with 3 efforts of 5 minutes each in Zone 4, alternating with 4-minute recoveries in Zone 2.

Maintenance

Test yourself again and see if you have improved to 2 stars, then follow that program.

If you are still at 1 star, repeat from Week 7 onward.

IF YOU HAVE 2 STARS:

You are below average. The first question we must ask is why? Do you deserve this score? If you are very healthy and don't exercise, it's important for you to learn and appreciate the value of exercise. The only thing between you and 3, 4, or 5 stars is your level of motivation. But if you walk every day, try to stay in the right weight range, and have focused on cardiovascular training, you may have a medical problem. A score this low is sometimes the result of a silent medical condition. It is best that you talk to your physician.

If your doctor approves of your beginning an exercise program, you need to choose an aerobic activity that is easy. Walking, swimming, and bike riding on flat roads are all good options. If you have musculoskeletal problems, such as bad knees, you may want to consider swimming, bicycle riding on flat roads, using an elliptical trainer if you have access to a gym, or swimming and aquaerobics if you have access to a pool.

As you work your way steadily through your exercise program, you must give your body time to adapt to the increasing effort. Remember, you have a lot of potential to improve.

Weeks 1–3

You will want to calendar:

- A walk, swim, or ride every second day or 3 to 4 days a week.
- Warm up for 10 minutes each day in Zone 1.
- Work out for 15 to 20 minutes in Zones 2 and 3.
- Slowly increase the number of minutes you spend in Zone 3, with at least equal time spent recovering in Zone 2.
- To improve, gradually increase your distance or intensity (speed) in small increments. But remember that the goal is not how long or how hard you go, it's that you are getting out and moving, and every time you move you do some good—you improve your cardiovascular and muscular fitness and increase your bone density.

Week 4

- Add one aerobic workout, so you are now doing 4 to 5.
- Warm up each time for 10 minutes in Zone 1.

- Increase one of the 4 to 5 workouts to 30 minutes in Zones 2 and 3 (alternating 4 minutes in Zone 3 with 2 minutes in Zone 2).
- To improve your aerobic capacity do one of the shorter, 20- to 25-minute days, at a higher intensity, in Zone 3 (alternating 6 minutes in Zone 3 with 2 minutes in Zone 2). You still need to warm up for 10 minutes before this workout.

Week 5

- This is a recovery week. Repeat one week from the program you used in Weeks 1–3.

Weeks 6–8

- Warm up each session for 10 minutes in Zone 1.
- Do 5 workouts per week, with two of 30 minutes each alternating 4 minutes in Zone 3 with 2 minutes in Zone 2.
- Do two of the 20–25-minute workouts a little faster, alternating 8 minutes in Zone 3 with 2 minutes in Zone 2.
- Add one workout of 45 minutes in length, alternating 10 minutes in Zone 2 with 3 minutes in Zone 3 and 2 minutes in Zone 4.

Week 9

- Repeat Week 4.

Weeks 10–12

- Warm up each time for 10 minutes in Zone 1.
- Do 5 to 6 workouts per week.
- Do two 30-minute workouts, alternating 4 minutes in Zone 3 with 2 minutes in Zone 2.
- Do one or two 20-minute workouts, alternating 8 minutes in Zone 3 with 2 minutes in Zone 2.
- Do two 45-minute workouts, alternating 5 minutes in Zone 2 with 5 minutes in Zone 3 and 5 minutes in Zone 4.

Maintenance

Test yourself again and see if you now score 3 stars. If so, continue using the 3-star program. If not, repeat the 2-star program from Week 6 onward, and then test your aerobic score again. Hopefully you will show improvement on the walking test.

IF YOU SCORED 3 STARS:

If you have no physical limitations, you may choose from among the aerobic activities listed on page 231.

Weeks 1–4

To maintain or improve your aerobic training level, you need to calendar:

- 3 to 6 sessions of aerobic training per week.
- Always warm up for 10 minutes in Zone 1 before each workout.
- 2 to 3 times per week work out for 20 to 30 minutes in Zones 2 and 3 (alternating 5 minutes in Zone 3 with 5 minutes in Zone 2).
- Twice per week enjoy a longer workout (45 to 60 minutes) in Zones 2 and 3.
- Week 4: This is your recovery week. This will give your body time to rest and gain strength for the next cycle. This is not a waste of time. Recovery is as important as the hardest training week. Remember, improvements happen during recovery! Train only 3 times, without performing the longer workout.

Weeks 5–8

- Calendar 3 to 5 sessions of aerobic training per week.
- Always warm up for 10 minutes in Zone 1 before your workout.
- 2 to 3 times per week work out for 40 to 50 minutes in Zones 2 and 3 (alternating 6 minutes in Zone 3 with 4 minutes in Zone 2).
- Once per week perform some interval training breaking into Zone 4 (alternating 3 minutes in Zone 4 with 2 minutes in Zone 2) for a total of 20 minutes.

- Twice per week enjoy a longer workout (50 to 60 minutes) in Zones 2 and 3, gradually increasing the time in Zone 3. In the middle, go into Zone 4 for 10 minutes.
- At Week 6, if you feel your workouts are getting easy and that you are progressing quickly, retest. If you've advanced to 4 stars, in Week 7 start at Week 1 in the 4-star program and follow the first six weeks of that program for your remaining six weeks.
- Week 8: Train only 3 times, without performing the longer workout.

Weeks 9–12

- Schedule 4 to 5 sessions of aerobic training per week.
- Always warm up for 10 minutes in Zone 1 before your workout.
- 1 to 2 times per week work out for 40 to 60 minutes in Zones 2 and 3 (alternating 6 to 8 minutes in Zone 3 with 2 to 4 minutes in Zone 2).
- Twice per week perform some interval training breaking into Zone 4 (alternating 4 minutes in Zone 4 with 2 minutes in Zones 2 and 3) for a total of 20 to 30 minutes.
- Twice per week enjoy a longer workout (50 to 60 minutes) in Zones 2 and 3, gradually increasing the time in Zone 3. In the middle, go into Zone 4 for 10 minutes.

Maintenance

- Work out aerobically 4 to 6 times per week, 30 to 60 minutes per session. Warm up and recover Zones 1 and 2.
- Alternate 45- to 60-minute training sessions with efforts in Zones 2 and 3, with 20- to 30-minute sessions including interval training in Zone 4. Gradually increase working time, until you feel comfortable doing 4 to 6 sessions of an hour each every week.
- Every 2 to 3 weeks have an easier week, with only 3 to 4 workouts. Reduce your training volume by 10 to 15 percent during your easy week.

IF YOU SCORED 4 STARS:

If you have no physical limitations you may select from among the activities listed on page 231.

You are above average. You don't have to worry about your cardiovascular fitness, but we all want to improve. Here is an aerobic program that will help you to do just that.

Weeks 1–4

- Calendar 3 to 5 sessions of aerobic training per week.
- Always warm up for 10 minutes in Zone 1 before your workout.
- 2 to 3 times per week work out for 30 to 40 minutes in Zones 2 and 3 (alternating 5 minutes in Zone 3 with 2 to 3 minutes in Zone 2).
- 1 to 2 times per week perform some interval training breaking into Zone 4 (alternating 3 minutes in Zone 4 with 5 minutes in Zones 2 and 3) for a total of 15 to 30 minutes.
- 1 to 2 times per week enjoy a longer workout (45 to 60 minutes) in Zones 2 and 3, gradually increasing the time in Zone 3. In the middle, go into Zone 4 for 10 minutes.
- Week 4: This is your recovery week. This will give your body time to rest and gain strength for the next cycle. This is not a waste of time. Recovery is as important as the hardest training week. Remember, improvements happen during recovery! Train only 3 times, without performing any longer workout.

Weeks 5–8

- Calendar 3 to 5 sessions of aerobic training per week.
- Always warm up for 10 minutes in Zone 1 before your workout.
- 2 times per week, work out for 40 to 50 minutes in Zones 2 and 3, alternating 6 minutes in Zone 3 with 2 to 3 minutes in Zone 2.
- 2 times per week perform some interval training breaking into Zone 4 (alternating 3 to 5 minutes in Zone 4 with 3 minutes in Zones 2 and 3) for a total of 15 to 30 minutes.
- Once per week, enjoy a longer workout (50 to 70 minutes) in Zones 2

and 3, gradually increasing the time in Zone 3. In the middle, go into Zone 4 for 10 minutes.

- At Week 6, if you feel your workouts are getting easy and that you are progressing quickly, retest. If you've advanced to 5 stars, in Week 7 start at Week 1 in the 5-star program and follow the first 6 weeks of that program for your remaining 6 weeks.
- Week 8: Train only 3 times, with two workouts in Zones 2 and 3, and only one interval training day.

Weeks 9–12

- Calendar 3 to 6 sessions of aerobic training per week.
- Always warm up for 10 to 15 minutes in Zone 1 before your workout.
- 2 times per week, work out for 60 minutes in Zones 2 and 3 (alternating 8 to 10 minutes in Zone 3, with 3 to 4 minutes in Zone 2).
- 2 times per week perform some interval training breaking into Zone 4 (alternating 5 minutes in Zone 4 with 2 to 3 minutes in Zones 2 and 3) for a total of 20 to 40 minutes.
- Twice per week enjoy a longer workout (60 to 75 minutes) in Zones 2 and 3, gradually increasing the time in Zone 3. Every 15 minutes, break into Zone 4 and hold it for 5 to 8 minutes.

Maintenance

- Exercise between 3 and 6 times a week.
- Try to build workouts to around or over an hour.
- Over time, when that becomes easy, increase intensity by adding more time in Zones 3 and 4.
- You can start building time into Zone 4, from 5 minutes up to 10 to 15 minutes. For these Zone 4 efforts, keep recovery time equal to 50 percent of your working time.
- Every 2 to 3 weeks, have an easier week, with only 3 to 4 workouts. Reduce your training volume by 10 to 15 percent during your easy week.

IF YOU SCORED 5 STARS:

If you have no physical limitations you may select from among the activities listed on page 231.

You are already in good aerobic shape. You can keep doing what you are already doing, if you like. If you are competing, you need to dedicate most of your time to training modalities that are specific to your discipline. If you are just looking to stay in shape, using cross-training, here are some ideas.

Weeks 1–4

To maintain your fitness level, you will want to calendar:

- 3 to 5 sessions of your aerobic training per week.
- Always warm up for 10 minutes in Zone 1 before your workout.
- 1 to 3 times per week work out for 30 to 40 minutes in Zones 2 and 3, alternating 6 to 8 minutes in Zone 3, with 2 minutes in Zone 2.
- 1 to 2 times per week perform some interval training breaking into Zone 4 (alternating 3 to 5 minutes in Zone 4 with 3 to 5 minutes in Zones 2 and 3) for a total of 15 to 30 minutes.
- 1 to 2 times per week enjoy a longer workout (60 to 90 minutes) in Zones 2 and 3.
- Week 4: This is your recovery week. This will give your body time to rest and gain strength for the next cycle. This is as important as the hardest training week. Remember, improvements happen during recovery! Train 3 to 4 times, without the longer days.

Weeks 5–8

- Calendar 3 to 6 sessions of aerobic training per week.
- Always warm up for 10 to 15 minutes in Zone 1 before your workout.
- 1 to 3 times per week work out for 30 to 50 minutes in Zones 2 and 3, alternating 4 to 8 minutes in Zone 3, with 1 to 2 minutes in Zone 2.
- 1 to 2 times per week perform some interval training breaking into Zone 4 (alternate 3 to 5 minutes in Zone 4 with 2 to 3 minutes in Zones 2 and 3), for a total of 15 to 30 minutes.

- Once per week perform some sprint intervals. Alternate 15 seconds of high intensity (≈90 percent of your max) with 40 to 60 seconds of recovery at an easy intensity. Perform 2 sets of 3 to 4 minutes, with 3 to 5 minutes rest in between.
- Once per week enjoy a longer workout (60 to 90 minutes) in Zones 2 and 3, with 10 minutes in Zone 4 in the middle.
- Week 8: Recovery week. Train 3 to 4 times, with 2 to 3 workouts in Zones 2 and 3, and 1 interval training day.

Weeks 9–12

- Calendar 4 to 6 sessions of aerobic training per week.
- Always warm up for 10 to 15 minutes in Zones 1 and 2 before your workout.
- 1 to 2 times per week work out for 40 to 60 minutes in Zones 2 and 3, alternating 8 minutes in Zone 3, with 2 minutes in Zone 2.
- 2 times per week perform some interval training breaking into Zone 4 (alternating 3 minutes in Zone 4 with 3 minutes in Zones 2 and 3) for a total of 20 to 30 minutes.
- Once per week perform some sprint intervals. Alternate 15 seconds of high intensity with 45 seconds of recovery at an easy intensity. Perform 3 sets of 5 minutes, with 3-minute rests in between.
- Once per week enjoy a longer workout (60 to 90 minutes), in Zones 2 and 3, with 15 minutes in Zone 4 in the middle.

Maintenance

As we mentioned, you may already be a competitive athlete. If you're currently training three days or fewer a week, you are gifted. Try increasing to five or six days per week, but no more than six. Always allow one day for recovery. Add more interval training or high-intensity reps to your workout. To improve further, you need to be more specific. If your purpose is to compete, your needs go beyond the purpose of this book. You need training methodology specific to your sport. We are planning to dedicate future books to competitive training in different sports like cycling, running, and triathlon, but for now you need to seek advice elsewhere.

■ Every 2 to 3 weeks, have an easier week, with only 3 to 4 workouts. Reduce your training volume by 10 to 15 percent during your easy week.

Suitable Aerobic Activities

■ walking
■ running
■ cycling
■ jumping rope
■ stair climbing
■ Spinning
■ dance
■ elliptical ergometer
■ StairMaster
■ treadmill
■ aerobic circuit training (five minutes each on a stationary bike, treadmill, elliptical, Stairmaster, for two circuits)
■ swimming
■ step or water aerobics
■ riding a stationary bike
■ Jazzercise
■ Frisbee
■ golf (if you walk fast between holes)
■ basketball
■ soccer
■ more

But activity does not have to occur at a gym or in workout clothes to yield a bounty healthwise. Actively playing with children, scrubbing the floor, mowing the lawn, raking, pushing a lawn mower, and washing or waxing a car count as well. The Centers for Disease Control considers the following activities as effective aerobic activities (listed in ascending order from those activities that are less vigorous but require more time to be effective, to those that are more vigorous but require less time):

■ washing and waxing a car for 45 to 60 minutes
■ washing windows or floors for 45 to 60 minutes

- playing volleyball for 45 minutes
- playing touch football for 30 to 45 minutes
- gardening for 30 to 45 minutes
- wheeling self in wheelchair for 30 to 40 minutes
- walking 1¾ miles in 35 minutes (20 min/mile)
- basketball (shooting baskets) for 30 minutes
- bicycling 5 miles in 30 minutes
- dancing fast (social) for 30 minutes
- pushing a stroller 1½ miles in 30 minutes
- raking leaves for 30 minutes
- walking 2 miles in 30 minutes (15 min/mile)
- water aerobics for 30 minutes
- swimming laps for 20 minutes
- wheelchair basketball for 20 minutes
- basketball (playing a game) for 15 to 20 minutes
- bicycling 4 miles in 15 minutes
- jumping rope for 15 minutes
- running 1½ miles in 15 minutes (10 min/mile)
- shoveling snow for 15 minutes
- stair walking for 15 minutes

Flexibility

Flexibility is a staple to fitness. Our level of flexibility is not fixed, as conventional wisdom dictates, but can—and should—be improved to aid in a long, healthy, and functional life. Scientifically, word is still out whether improving flexibility prevents injury, but clearly stretching packs a punch with regard to everyday living. With increased flexibility, every move you make is easier: putting on your socks, sitting on an airplane or in the backseat of a car, or reaching a higher cupboard.

One of the best professional cyclists I have coached, Andy Hampsten, was very dedicated to stretching. He committed a significant amount of time to it. Every single day—even the very most important day of the Giro d'Italia or Tour de France—he'd be doing his flexibility exercises. He traveled with a little mattress and even at the airport I'd see him doing his flexibility exercises.

> Andy knew that he could have more energy to spend on exercise if he didn't waste power stretching tight muscles and tendons with every pedal stroke. As a result he could translate tremendous power to the pedals because he didn't have much internal resistance to overcome.
>
> —Max

Think of your muscles as dough. Stretching exercises increase your muscle temperature. As your muscles get warmer, they become more pliable and flexible. Stretching leads to longer muscles, which give you greater range of motion.

Stretching and flexibility activities you may enjoy at any level include yoga, Pilates, and traditional static stretching. (See pages 242 to 248 for two stretching routines we supply to our athletes.) Many people enjoy taking time to do yoga or Pilates on their own. For them it is a time to relax, put on music, breathe. Some prefer a scheduled class led by a knowledgeable instructor. If you are not flexible, you may not like flexibility class to start with, but keep with it—along with an easier time in class you will gain additional mobility in your everyday life. Whether it's your first class or your fiftieth, always go at your own pace. And remember, don't stretch when you are cold. If you try to stretch cold muscles, your muscles will tighten. Warm up by jogging in place or walking around the block first.

To establish a flexibility starting point that takes mitigating factors into account, we offer the Sit and Reach test to assess your flexibility.

The Sit and Reach test is a classic flexibility test, since it's easy, it doesn't require expensive equipment, and it takes little time. This test explores your ability to flex forward from a seated position. It doesn't measure the flexibility or the range of motion of all of your joints; it mainly tests the flexibility of your hamstrings and back muscles. It also relies on the strength of your abdomen and hip flexors. All of these elements contribute to your score. For a more precise evaluation of your flexibility, you can see a physical therapist or a fitness instructor.

Also note that because this test measures how close the tips of your fingers get to your toes, it gives a bonus to people with short legs and a long torso or with strong abdominal muscles, and it dings people with long legs and a short torso—even if you do yoga and can fold yourself in half like a book. If you have long legs your fingertips are not going to get too close to your toes. Despite these caveats, it measures your current flexibility and will be accurate in tracking your improvement.

Sit and Reach Test

- Place a line of tape 15 inches long on the floor.
- Place a yardstick or extended tape measure perpendicular to the tape to form a T, with the 15-inch mark of the yardstick intersecting the tape.
- Warm up briefly, then sit on the floor with your shoes off, legs extended.
- Place your feet 10 to 12 inches apart with your heels on the tape *and the 0-inch end* of the ruler between your knees.
- Place one hand over your other hand and reach as far as possible over the ruler without bending your knees.
- Note the inch mark on the ruler you are able to touch with your fingertips.

Using the best of three tries, score yourself 1 to 5 stars.

If you scored:

1 star: Your flexibility score is definitely low. If you also have a history of back or joint pain, you should talk with your health-care provider or physical therapist regarding whether or not you have a condition that is hindering your flexibility. You also need to approach fitness carefully. The good news is that you have the greatest potential for improvement. Improving your flexibility will bring considerable quality back into your life.

2 stars: You're definitely stiff. You need some stretching in your life. So take advantage of the stretching program.

3 stars: You have average flexibility. You can do better and will feel better for it.

4 stars: You are above average. If you have never stretched and your performance is just the result of natural flexibility, you'll want to rule out a possible hypermobility condition. Talk to your doctor. If you have been stretching or taking yoga classes, you have been taking good care of your flexibility. However, there is still room for improvement.

5 stars: Yoga instructor! Seriously, good job. Whatever you are currently doing is working. Just make sure you don't have hypermobility problems.

FEMALE NORMS FOR THE SIT AND REACH TEST
(NUMBER OF INCHES)

RATINGS	AGE (years)							
	18-25	26-35	36-45	45-55	56-65	66-75	76-85	86-95
★★★★★	>23	>26	>21	>20	>19	>19	?	?
★★★★	>19	>17	>17	>15	>13	>13	?	?
★★★	17-18	15-16	15-16	13-14	11-12	10-12	?	?
★★	14-16	13-14	13-14	10-12	9-10	8-9	?	?
★	<13	<12	<12	<9	<8	<7	?	?

MALE NORMS FOR THE SIT AND REACH TEST
(NUMBER OF INCHES)

RATINGS	AGE (years)							
	18-25	26-35	36-45	45-55	56-65	66-75	76-85	86-95
★★★★★	>21	>19	>19	>18	>14-15	>14-15	?	?
★★★★	>21	>20	>19	>18	>17	>17	?	?
★★★	19-20	19	17-18	16-17	15-16	15-16	?	?
★★	17-18	16-18	15-16	14-15	13-14	13-14	?	?
★	<16	<15	<14	<13	<12	<12	?	?

Basic instructions for all levels:

- At the end of this section, you will find the A and B stretching exercises referred to in the instructions.
- Stretch only until you feel a light stretching of the muscle, not pain. Any sensation of pain will trigger contraction of the muscles you are trying to stretch.

Useful tips:

- Wear loose comfy clothing.
- To facilitate stretching, warm up your muscles beforehand by taking a hot shower or begin with easy movements.

- Start by stretching the muscles in your hands, wrists, arms, and shoulders first, and then proceed to stretching your neck, back, trunk, hips, and lower extremities.
- Don't hold your breath while stretching.
- When stretching a muscle that goes over two joints—say, the muscle that starts above your knee and attaches to the Achilles tendon on your heel, it's better to stretch the two joints separately.
- Gentle, longer stretches are more effective; you have to get longer gradually.
- Massage and relaxation techniques can be used to enhance stretching.

Do *not* stretch if:

- You do not have full range of motion in that particular joint.
- You have a fracture (you may think you are losing time waiting for the injury to heal and want to stretch the joint, but stretching applies stress to the line of fracture and actually slows healing).
- You have swelling, which is an acute inflammatory response. This indicates the muscle is healing. What is normally a gentle stress such as stretching can cause tremendous stress during this time.
- You have very loose joints or can overextend the joint (such as hyperextending your knees), or the joint is excessively slack. Excessive laxity can be congenital, or due to a recent or past injury, such as a torn ligament. Part of the joint's current stability could be the result of muscle rigidity. If you stretch the muscle or make it suppler, you could lose that stability.

If you experience pain, discomfort, or difficulties in reaching and/or holding the positions, talk to your health-care provider or physical therapist.

To boost your flexibility as much as possible, space your flexibility workouts as follows:

- Always stretch religiously before each muscular-strengthening and aerobic session you do.
- Schedule your specific flexibility sessions on the same days you do muscular-strengthening work or light aerobic work.

- Schedule flexibility rest days on the days you do hard aerobic training. Combining days you do flexibility and strength training is fine.

IF YOU SCORED 1 STAR:

Set up a meeting with your health-care provider or a physical therapist and have her assess whether or not you have any musculoskeletal conditions that may be causing this. If you get the green light, start very easy. You need more warm-up prior to stretching than others. Increasing your body and muscle temperature is a way to make your muscles and joints more flexible. Try a warm bath or shower before stretching. Also walk or ride a stationary bike prior to stretching. Your priority is to avoid making things worse, so be careful.

Weeks 1–4

- Start with the A exercises on pages 242–4, 3 times a week. Your goal for these first four weeks is to get familiar with the stretching positions. Focus on that. Try to understand how much your body can do. You don't have to reach the final position if it feels too hard. You can make things easier by using a towel or a stretching band when performing some of the exercises. Avoid jerky movements.
- Do not stretch when you are cold. Warm up by walking around the block or using a treadmill or stationary bike. If you try to stretch cold muscles, your muscles will tighten because of the stretch reflex.
- Exhale and relax as you reach each position.
- Hold every position for just 10 to 15 seconds.
- Again, do with your mind what you're trying to do with your muscles: relax.
- Listen to the degree of tension in your body. You may perhaps feel a little discomfort; this is okay. But do not push yourself to the point of pain. If you reach pain, your muscles will contract and stiffen more.

Weeks 5–8

- Continue with your stretching routine. You can increase to four times a week.

- Increase the length of your routine by adding a second stretch of 15 to 20 seconds for each position.

Weeks 9–12

Now you should be able to stretch 5 times a week.

- Keep performing the A exercises.
- Exhale and relax as you reach each position.
- Hold every position for 20 to 30 seconds 2 times.
- Again, do with your mind what you're trying to do with your muscles: relax.
- Listen to the degree of tension in your body. You may perhaps feel a little discomfort; this is okay. But do not push yourself to the point of pain. If you reach pain, your muscles with contract and stiffen more.
- At the end of this block, redo the sit and reach test. Hopefully you are getting better!

IF YOU SCORED 2 STARS:

You are definitely stiff. You need to dedicate time to stretching in order to regain your flexibility and all of the quality of life that goes with it. However, you need to be cautious in starting your program.

Weeks 1–4

- Start with the A exercises on pages 242–4 3 to 4 times a week.
- Do not stretch when you are cold. Warm up by jogging in place or walking around the block. If you try to stretch cold muscles, your muscles will tighten because of the stretch reflex.
- Exhale and relax as you reach each position.
- Hold every position for 15 to 20 seconds.
- Again, do with your mind what you're trying to do with your muscles: relax.
- Listen to the degree of tension in your body. You may perhaps feel a little discomfort; this is okay. But do not push yourself to the point of pain. If you reach pain, your muscles will contract and stiffen more.

Weeks 5–8

- Continue with your stretching routine.
- Increase the length of time by adding a second stretch of 20 to 30 seconds for each position.
- Increase the frequency to 5 times a week.

Weeks 9–12

- If you are tolerating the routine better, and it actually feels easy, add the B exercises on pages 245–8.
- At the end of this four-week block, redo the sit and reach test. Hopefully you can move up to the 3-star level.

IF YOU SCORED 3 STARS:

You are average. Incorporating more stretching into your life will give you greater flexibility and better overall health and mobility. If you are already stretching, and are in an improvement phase, look at the stretching exercises A and B on pages 242–8, and adopt anything you are not currently doing.

You can increase the benefits of your routine by adding new stretching exercises and/or by increasing the time you stretch every week (we favor five days a week). You can also increase the time you hold each position or increase the number of repetitions you perform, but stop if the stretch becomes painful or uncomfortable.

If you are not stretching yet, the good news is that you can become very good at flexibility.

Weeks 1–4

- Calendar stretching at least every second day of the week or—even better—five times a week.
- Perform the A exercises on pages 242–4.
- Do not stretch when you are cold. Warm up by jogging in place or walking around the block. If you try to stretch cold muscles, your muscles will tighten because of the stretch reflex.

- Exhale and relax as you reach each position.
- Hold every position for 15 to 30 seconds.
- Again, do with your mind what you're trying to do with your muscles: relax.
- Listen to the degree of tension in your body. You may perhaps feel a little discomfort; this is okay. But do not push yourself to the point of pain. If you reach pain, your muscles will contract and stiffen more.

Weeks 5–8

- Continue with your routine of stretching every other day or 5 times a week.
- Add the B exercises on pages 245–8.
- 1 or 2 times a week, stretch twice a day.
- Increase the length of time you hold each position to 30 seconds 2 times.

Weeks 9–12

- Redo the sit and reach test. If you score 4 to 5 stars now, move up to the instructions for that score. If you are still 3 stars, increase the frequency of your stretching routine by one or two more times a week. You can also add some different stretching modalities, such as dynamic (ballistic) stretching or Proprioceptive Neuromuscular Facilitation (PNF). This technique involves a short muscular contraction (5 to 10 seconds) before stretching the muscle 10 to 20 seconds, to be repeated 2 to 3 times. PNF stretching is very easy when you have the help of a partner. First, mildly stretch the muscle group you are targeting for 15 to 20 seconds. At this point, contract the muscle for 5 to 10 seconds, while your partner is resisting the movement you are trying to perform. Mild force should be applied to avoid injury. Immediately after you relax the muscle, your partner should gently stretch it for 20 to 30 seconds. Rest for 30 seconds and repeat.

However, keep in mind that the main goal of your training is not for you to simply score more stars but for you to feel better. We have patients who never score very high in the sit and reach test (perhaps they just have long legs and a short torso), but they still do extremely well in getting stronger, faster, and better.

IF YOU SCORED 4 OR 5 STARS:

You are doing well. You are probably already taking classes or stretching regularly. No? Then you can consider adding Pilates or yoga classes to your week to maintain this level of flexibility as you age. Taking classes makes flexibility work more interesting and effective. If you prefer to train by yourself and use flexibility exercises as a moment to enjoy your own time to relax and reduce anxiety, look at the exercises at the end of this section on page 249. Keep in mind that there is not only one way to gain fitness, so if you want to stay with your current program, do so. Your good score just validated it.

Weeks 1–12

Since you are already doing very well, you don't have to follow a particular progression in increasing your stretching routine. Just find the sequence of exercises you enjoy more, and make it your lifelong anti-stiffness medicine.

If you want to follow our routine, do the following:

We recommend stretching daily, but at least 5 days a week.

- Perform all of the stretching exercises A and B on pages 242–8.
- Stretch gently to the illustrated position. Exhale while reaching each position. Hold each position for 15 to 20 seconds, breathing regularly.
- You should experience a sensation of a light stretch of the muscles, without pain. When the muscles get used to the position, increase the stretch a bit, and hold for another 15 to 20 seconds.

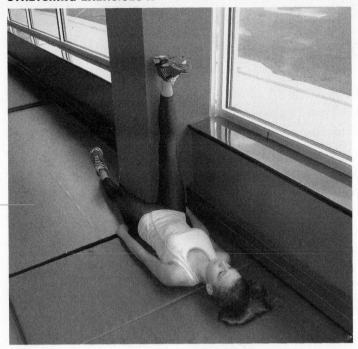

Door frame stretch: Lying on your back with one leg resting along the vertical frame of the door and your buttocks against the baseboard, keep your back flat. The opposite leg should lie straight on the floor. A right angle should be made between your two legs. Hold sixty seconds on each side, twice. This exercise mainly stretches your hamstrings and glutes.

Calves: With both feet facing forward and your front leg bent at the knee, lean forward using your arms for support against a wall, until you feel the stretch on the calf of your rear leg. Keep your upper body well aligned. This exercise stretches your gastrocnemius, a two-joint muscle that originates above your knee. It works as a plantar flexor (allowing you to rise on your toes) or as a knee flexor.

Repeat with your rear leg slightly bent at the knee. This exercise stretches the soleus, a plantar flexor that crosses only one joint, the ankle.

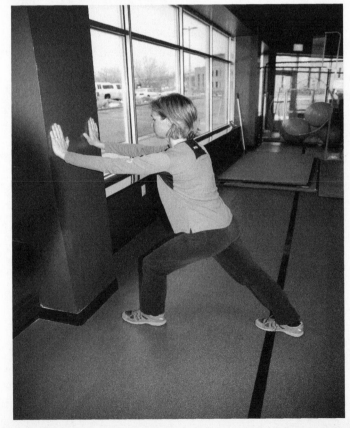

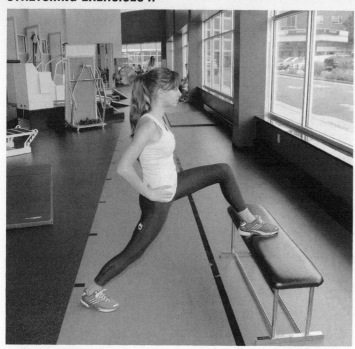

Hip flexors using a chair. Keep one leg forward, with your foot on a chair or bench as illustrated. Your rear leg should be slightly bent at the knee. Keep your upper body straight. You should feel this stretch in the upper thigh of your rear leg.

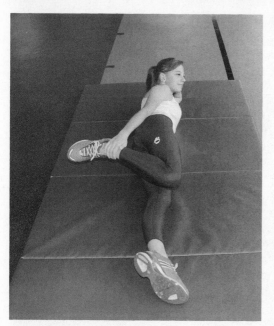

Lying quads: Hold one foot behind your back as illustrated. Keep your leg parallel to the floor.

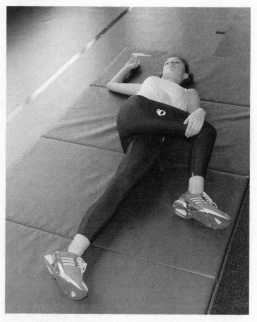

Pectoral, oblique, and hip external rotators: Lying on your back, keep your shoulders on the floor, and bend your hip and knee at ninety degrees. Bring the bent knee across your midline and over the opposite leg, which is relaxed on the floor. Rest your hand on the opposite side of your bent knee. While staying in this relaxed position, bend your same side arm at a ninety-degree angle at the elbow as illustrated.

STRETCHING EXERCISES A

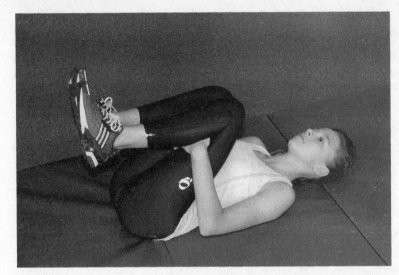

Low back and glutes: Lying down on your back, bring your knees to your chest. Place your hands on the back side of your knee and gently press your thighs against your chest as illustrated.

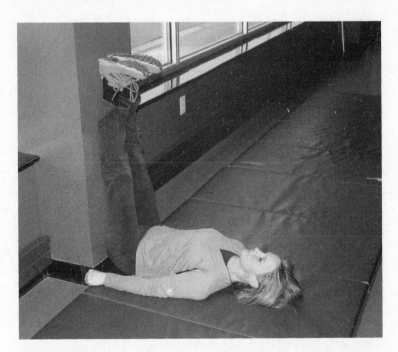

Legs against the wall. Keep both legs straight against the wall, at approximately a ninety-degree angle to your upper body. Keep your back flat. This exercise stretches all the posterior chain (back, lumbar fascia, glutes, hamstrings). Hold for 3 to 5 minutes. If your feet get numb or tingle, hold the position for less time.

STRETCHING EXERCISES B

Hamstring stretch: Facing a bench, place one leg on the bench with your foot flexed. Slowly bend forward over your leg. Place your hands on your lower back as shown.

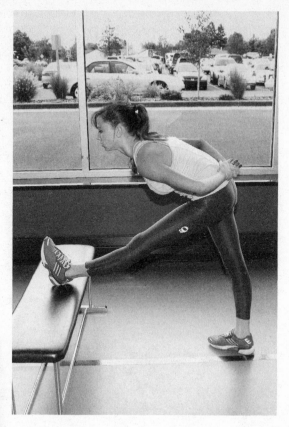

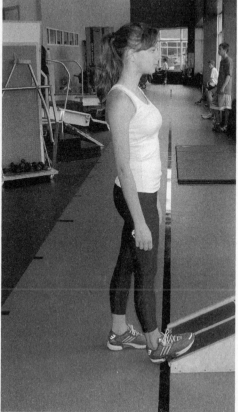

Standing calves stretch with step: Place your foot diagonal to a step, with your heel touching the floor. Hold the stretch with your arms at your sides.

Hip flexors lunge on floor: Standing straight, lunge forward toward the ground using your arms for support. Rest your back knee on the mat. Your front knee should be positioned above your front heel with your toes facing forward. Regulate the degree of stretch by sliding your rear leg forward or back. Make sure that the heel of your rear leg is pointing up, and both legs are parallel to each other.

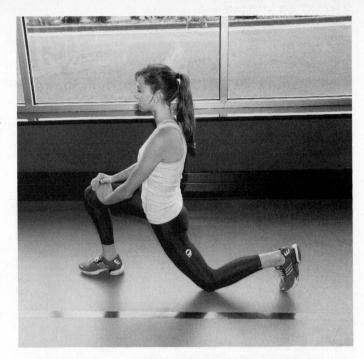

Vertical quad stretch: Using a wall for support, pull your leg back toward your buttocks. Grasp your leg at the ankle with your free hand.

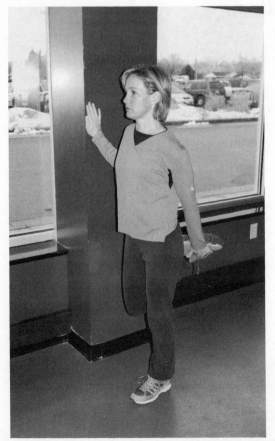

STRETCHING EXERCISES B

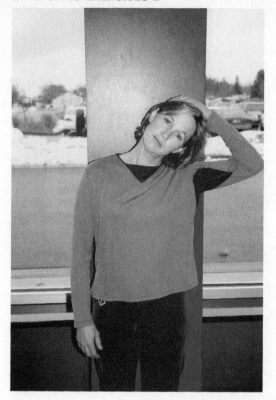

Upper trapezius stretch: Sitting or standing in an upright position, place one arm bent at the elbow behind your back or hanging straight at your side. With the other hand resting on the opposite side of your head above the ear, gently pull down toward your shoulder. Make sure your face is always looking forward.

ITB, hip external rotators: Lying on your back, bring both legs up at a ninety-degree angle at your hip and knee. Cross one foot in front of the opposite knee as illustrated. Using both hands, gently pull your opposite knee toward your chest.

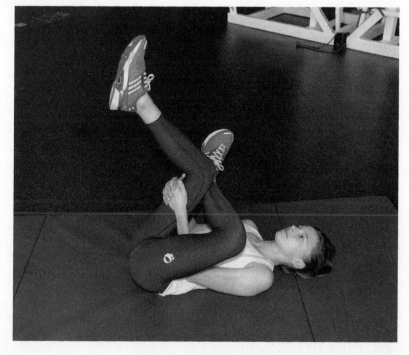

STRETCHING EXERCISES B

Lateral rotation against wall: Stand next to a wall, with your foot closer to the wall forward. Rotate your upper body to face the wall, with the arm and shoulder closer to the wall extended. Press this arm against the wall, keeping your hand at the same height as your shoulder as illustrated.

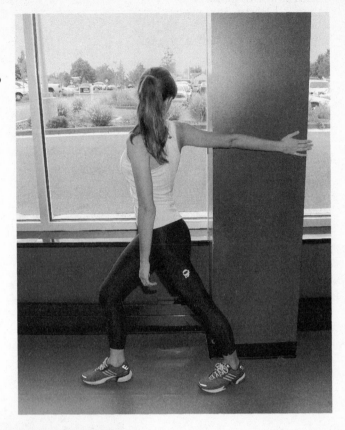

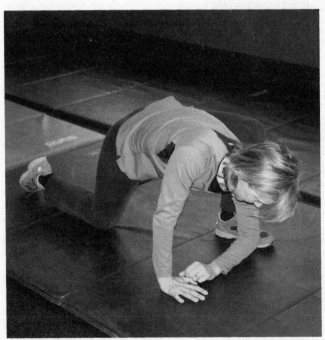

Hip flexors, lower back combo: Kneel down on the mat. The foot of one leg and the knee of the other leg should be resting on the mat. If your right knee is resting, then place your right hand on the mat straight down from your shoulder as illustrated. Place your left hand near the thumb of your right hand and slowly try to touch the mat with your left elbow, at about the arch of your left foot. You can slide your right leg back and forth to find the appropriate stretch. Do the same stretch with the opposite leg forward.

Suitable flexibility activities include:

- gymnastics
- dancing
- climbing
- yoga
- skipping rope
- stretching
- Pilates
- ballet
- water workouts
- Tai Chi
- other martial arts
- range of motion activities
- exercise with elastic tubing or a balance ball

Muscular Strength

Never fear, we are not going to try to turn you into a power lifter. Nor do you have to adopt a fondness for barbells and dumbbells. On the contrary, improved muscular strength benefits you in ways that go far beyond bulging biceps, and you can gain muscular strength a number of ways.

Increased muscle strength prevents muscle aches and joint injuries, and research shows that weight lifting fights osteopenia (a term for bone mineral density that is lower than normal peak but not low enough to be classified as osteoporosis). Scientists have also proven that lifting decreases interabdominal fat, which also reduces the risk of heart disease.

Depending on how many repetitions and how much you load each repetition, you trigger your muscles to change in different ways. Each option we will offer is designed to develop your muscular endurance, power, and muscle strength. But you will focus on different techniques, depending on your muscular-strength score and your goals.

In designing your program, you will choose muscle-strengthening exercises that can be done at a gym, at home, or at work during a break. For muscular-strength exercise in a gym, for example, we offer various workouts, including circuit training using different machines with a set of repetitions at a variety of stations so that you are never triggering the same muscle two times in a row.

How you perform muscular strengthening depends on your goals. In general, you develop muscular strength if you lift a weight that is close (70 percent or more) to the maximum amount you could lift once. (More on how to determine this later.) The amount of weight you can lift only once is referred to as your one-repetition maximum (1RM). When you lift weight above 70 percent of your 1RM, you are developing muscular strength. If you are doing numerous repetitions using a weight or load that is below 30 to 40 percent of your 1RM, you are basically doing an aerobic workout that develops muscular endurance.

The Weight You Should Lift

Without having to perform your maximum effort, you can estimate your maximum strength in a manner that is precise enough to start. We never ask our clients to determine their 1RM by actually lifting 100 percent of it. Maximum lifting of that kind makes sense for power or competitive lifters, but not for the purpose of making you better and stronger while respecting your body and health. Instead, we recommend you estimate your 100 percent by lifting much less. Here's how.

Start with a weight that seems friendly. Lift it. Count how many times you can lift it easily.

If you can lift it easily and smoothly ten times, you are probably working at 75 to 80 percent of your maximum or one-repetition maximum (1RM).

15 times=50 percent of your 1RM

6 times=85–90 percent of your 1RM

In other words, if you try to lift fifty pounds and you can lift it five or six times, most likely you are working about 90 percent of your max, so your 1RM is probably fifty-five to fifty-six pounds. If you can lift it fifteen times? Your 1RM is around 100.

Once you have a sense of your strength, progress by five-pound increments. When you reach a point where you cannot control the motion and lift in good form, you're using too much weight. Here again, "no pain, no gain" is wrong—if you lift too much weight you will not only *not* enjoy the benefits of lifting but will also risk injury. If you cannot control the motion in good form, you have too much weight.

If you want to build muscle:

You will want to pump 8 to 12 repetitions at around 75 percent of your one-repetition maximum, with 1 to 3 minutes of recovery time in between.

If you want to lose weight:

You should use light weights, doing what we call super sets: three sets or more of 25 to 50 repetitions at a fast speed of contraction, with a short recovery between 1 to 1.5 minutes.

If you want to build strength and endurance:

Between these extremes there is a continuum of benefit that more or less develops strength versus endurance. The speed of contraction is very important in determining how your muscles change and improve. When you try to lift a weight that is close to your maximum, the speed of contraction you can develop is slow, so the power you are producing is not very high (remember, power equals force times speed). On the other hand, when you lift a weight around 60 to 70 percent of your maximum, the speed of contraction you can develop is much higher, so even if you are using a lighter weight, the resulting power (weight × speed) you achieve is higher than in the previous example. This is why athletes who need to increase sustainable power more than maximum power spend significant time working at 60 to 70 percent of their 1RM, and focus on high speed of contraction.

Potential Weights

Lifting weight is not just something you do in a gym. Every time you challenge the gravitational acceleration force (lifting your kids, climbing a flight of stairs, or carrying your groceries), you are performing resistance training. We encourage you to seize every opportunity to safely do so as often as possible. However, benefits come only if you reach a load big enough to trigger adaptation in your muscles. To all our patients who are starting or intensifying a weight-training program, we also recommend core-strengthening classes, such as Pilates and yoga.

For muscular-strength building you can do any of the following:

- Use your body weight (in exercises such as crunches and push-ups).
- Use household objects.
- Use free weights (dumbbells and barbells).
- Use weight machines (including home models such as Nautilus, Boflex, or those at the gym).

To help you decide, consider the pros and cons of each type of strengthening exercise.

Using your body weight

In the dynamic modality (when muscle contraction happens together with joint movements) examples include:

- Squats, lunges, and step-ups target your lower body.
- Sit-ups develop your core strength.
- Chin-ups and push-ups work your upper body.

In isometric modality (when muscle contraction doesn't result in body movement, for example when holding a static body position), examples include:

- Various Pilates exercises, such as the frontal and lateral bridge to strengthen abdominal muscles.

Frontal bridge:

Lie on floor, facedown, keeping your pelvis off the floor, with your weight on your toes and your elbows bent.

Lateral bridge:

Lie on your side, with your elbow bent at ninety degrees. Lift and hold up your pelvis, with your weight on your lateral foot and elbow on the same side. Start by holding the position 15 to 20 seconds. Increase over time.

Pros (for both dynamic and isometric body-weight exercises):

- You can do it everywhere.
- It's very cheap.
- It trains your whole body and forces your stabilizer muscles to work.
- It affords a relatively good workout.
- There's little risk of injury if you know the proper technique.

Cons:

- It lacks specificity, it's hard to trigger a single muscle, unless you are knowledgeable about kinesiology.
- It offers limited benefits for more advanced athletes.
- It can be kind of boring.

Using household objects

(rolling a car tire, lifting a sandbag or cement, bench-pressing your child or grandchild)

Pros:

- It's free.
- Opportunities abound and you get work done while getting a workout.
- You can do it anywhere.
- It strengthens your entire body and is very good for your stabilizer or core muscles.

Cons:

- There is a risk of injury. Weight in household objects such as sandbags can shift quickly, requiring you to recruit muscle groups fast to avoid loss of balance, which can cause injury.
- It's difficult to gauge the amount of training you're getting.

Using free weights

(gear designed for weight-lifting purposes, such as barbells and dumbbells)

Pros:

- It's safe if you know the technique.
- You can train any muscle group.
- It stimulates your stabilizers or core muscles.
- You get impressive benefit from your efforts.
- You can easily monitor the training load progression.

Cons:

- There is expense involved, whether in purchasing weights or in joining a club that has them.
- If you don't know the technique, you can injure yourself.
- You have to be careful about not increasing the weight too quickly (people often feel stronger after a few sessions, then they add weight too quickly and they injure themselves).

Using weight machines

Pros:

- They ensure that you are lifting safely, by positioning your body correctly.
- Each machine is designed to stress a specific muscle or muscle groups.
- They make lifting easy for beginners.
- It's easy to monitor the training load.

Cons:

- There is generally cost involved, in either joining a gym or procuring home equipment.
- You are not reproducing natural movements; you gain strength but it's a strength that does not fully transfer to the complex muscular activity typical of some sports.
- Machines don't stress stabilizer muscles as much as free weights.

Other options

There are other options to improve your muscular strength: isometrics (other than using body weight), plyometrics, and elastic bands. We won't provide routines or exercises for these options, but they are viable weight-training choices and you may want to consider them, in which case you can explore them on your own. Here are the pros and cons of these modalities to consider:

Isometrics

Isometrics are exercises in which your muscle length and joint angle don't change, such as when pushing or pulling an immovable object.

Pros:

- You can do it anywhere.
- It's cheap.
- It's safe.

Cons:

- It doesn't train the ability of your muscle to contract and relax.
- It offers limited options in training different muscle groups.
- The improvement is not as dramatic as with dynamic lifting.
- It doesn't train coordination between muscles.
- It doesn't train the elastic quality of the muscle.
- It must be done at 50 percent of your max or more to get a training effect (less than that is like picking up a pencil—it does not cause overload).
- Strength gain is specific to the joint angle at which you perform the effort; it doesn't strengthen the entire range of motion.

Plyometrics

In plyometrics, when the muscle contracts from a stretched condition, which increases the power developed during the contraction. Typically, plyometrics involves explosive movements, such as jump rope, jumping on a trampoline, and so on, to develop muscular power.

Pros:

- It's cheap.
- You can do it just about anywhere.

- It can boost the degree of weight you are moving by many times your body weight, a great way to spike power, especially for explosive sports.
- It also heightens the speed of muscle contraction (improving the jump height of a basketball player, for example, or the quickness of a soccer player).
- The bouncing of your body and the impact on the ground increases bone density.

Cons:

- There's a risk of injury, especially in older people, who have less elasticity, and in those in the early phase of training.
- It's generally for advanced athletes.
- It must be accompanied by significant warm-up, as well as another form of resistance training.

Elastic bands

Elastic-band routines can be done using surgical tubing, old bike tires, or resistance bands designed for exercise.

Pros:

- It can be cheap.
- It's lightweight, easy to transport, and can be done just about anywhere.
- Its level of resistance increases with the degree of muscle contraction, which is physiologically important.
- Likewise, it adapts to the angle of the joint. As you pull it toward you, for example, the band gets harder to pull.
- It also requires control in the relaxation phase, which works your muscles differently, in what is called an eccentric modality.

Cons:

- It offers limited options for training all muscle groups.
- It's difficult to monitor training improvements.
- It's difficult to control the intensity of the effort.
- If the opposite end of the band is not firmly anchored, it can cause injury.

Making the Best Choice

Take advantage of every opportunity you have, based on what you like to do, your philosophy on how to use resources, and your desire to take advantage of technologies. As we've detailed, there are benefits and downsides to each modality. Weight machines are, in many ways, ideal because the machine holds your body in the right position and isolates the proper muscles. Research indicates that lifting free weights, however, exercises more muscles than weight machines. It also increases the development of the stabilizers in your body by forcing your body to hold itself in the correct alignment. While one arm is doing the lifting, for example, the muscles in your back, legs, abdomen, and so on are working to stabilize your body. And this creates greater overall core strength. This is important because you are only as strong as your weakest muscles. If you squat down to pick something up, for example, your glutes and quads (large muscles that get more work than your core muscles) are fine. It's the muscles in your back that will be the first to protest with pangs.

Muscle Soreness

In the early phase of muscle strengthening we all experience muscle soreness. To minimize this, it's important to lift on the easy side. Unlike aerobic activity, where you feel the effort while you are engaged in the activity, in muscle strengthening you won't feel it while you're lifting, but you will feel it twenty-four hours or more later. Doctors call this Delayed Onset of Muscle Soreness or DOMS. Avoid DOMS. If you're scheduled to do two sets but feel like you could do a third, *don't*. For maximum benefit, follow the training principle of graduality. Remember, no patience, no gain.

Muscular-Strength Tests

These are very simple tests. They are not scientific in terms of measuring the strength of a single muscle. Since they've been used for so long, it's easy to compare yourself to the rest of the population. You will gauge your muscular strength by seeing how many push-ups and sit-ups you can do.

Push-ups:

To do a correct and safe push-up, always warm up by walking, jumping rope, or walking stairs beforehand. Start by doing one or two push-ups to ensure your back is not bothering you and your shoulders, wrists, and elbows are fine.

Knee push-ups: We recommend these for women and beginners or people with low strength. Place your hands on the floor, wider than shoulder width apart. Bend your knees and place them on the floor to support some of your weight. Try to keep your back as straight as possible. Lower your shoulders to the floor.

Regular push-ups: Place your toes and hands on the floor. With your back straight, fully extend your arms, then lower yourself to the floor.

Count how many you can do without stopping. It doesn't matter how fast or slow you do them.

Find your score on the appropriate chart.

FEMALE NORMS FOR THE PUSH-UP TEST (NUMBER COMPLETED)

	AGE (years)				
RATINGS	20-29	30-39	40-49	50-59	60-69
★ ★ ★ ★ ★	>27	>26	>22	>16	>15
★ ★ ★ ★	>22-26	>21-25	>18-21	>13-15	>12-14
★ ★ ★	16-21	14-20	12-17	9-12	6-11
★ ★	11-15	10-13	7-11	3-8	2-5
★	<10	<9	<6	<2	<1

MALE NORMS FOR THE PUSH-UP TEST (NUMBER COMPLETED)

	AGE (years)				
RATINGS	20-29	30-39	40-49	50-59	60-69
★ ★ ★ ★ ★	>35	>29	>23	>18	>14
★ ★ ★ ★	>30-34	>24-28	>19-22	>14-17	>11-13
★ ★ ★	24-29	19-23	13-18	10-13	9-10
★ ★	18-23	14-18	10-12	7-9	6-7
★	<17	<13	<9	<6	<5

Sit-ups

To do a safe and correct sit-up, sit on the floor with your knees bent. Cross your arms over your chest so that each hand is touching the opposite shoulder. (If you put your hands behind your head it strains your neck.) Lift your shoulders five to ten inches from the ground by curling upward using your stomach muscles. Focus on bending your abdomen rather than lifting a straight torso. Keep your chin close to your chest. Don't go all the way up. (When people go all the way up, they tend to give a push halfway up and finish on momentum.)

To perform the test, do as follows:

Do as many sit-ups as you can in 1 minute without stopping. Check against the appropriate chart to score yourself.

Add your two scores together and divide by two. If you scored:

5 stars: You are obviously a strong person, maybe already lifting weights.

4 stars: You are above average.

3 stars: You are in the average range. It is up to you to move up on the chart.

1 Minute Sit-up Test (Men)

Age	18-25	26-35	36-45	46-55	56-65	65+
*****	>49	>45	>41	>35	>31	>28
****	39-49	35-45	30-41	25-35	21-31	19-28
***	35-38	31-34	27-29	22-24	17-20	15-18
**	25-34	22-30	17-26	13-21	9-16	7-14
*	<25	<22	<17	<9	<9	<7

1 Minute Sit-up Test (Women)

Age	18-25	26-35	36-45	46-55	56-65	65+
*****	>43	>39	>33	>27	>24	>23
****	33-43	29-39	23-33	18-27	13-24	14-23
***	29-32	25-28	19-22	14-17	10-12	11-13
**	18-28	13-24	7-18	5-13	3-9	2-10
*	<18	<20	<7	<5	<3	<2

2 stars: You are below average.

1 star: You definitely must include lifting weights in your routine in order to stay healthy, look better, and feel better.

The following program is designed to improve your muscular strength. (For more in-depth discussion on how this happens, see Chapter 4, "Better Strength.")

Basic instructions for all levels:

■ Select your weight-training modality from the pool of those detailed here: using your body weight, free weights, or weight machines. The best one for you is the one that is easiest for you to use.

■ Have a trainer or friend who is experienced with lifting show you the correct positions and the right technique. The YMCA and EXRX Web sites show proper weight lifting technique in slow motion video.

■ Breathe in while relaxing and breathe out when contracting. If you keep your mouth closed, and you hold your breath while contracting your muscles, you increase the pressure inside your abdomen and chest. This limits the return of blood to your heart. An effort like lifting requires *more* blood, which your cardiovascular system can only deliver when the blood return to your heart is good. Holding your breath while also doing strenuous upper body physical work (such as shoveling snow or weight lifting) causes an even bigger stress on your heart. Remember, breathing right is the basis for healthy exercising.

■ Be aware of the alignment of your body with respect to the weight you are lifting or the movement you are performing.

■ If you want to do your weight training in a certain order, you can start doing bigger muscle groups first (they fatigue later because they have more resources).

■ Alternate exercises where you pull with ones that require you push.

To make the best use of your muscular strength program, on your calendar space your strengthening workouts as follows:

■ Slot your hardest muscular-strengthening session two days after your total rest day. (You will do aerobic exercise the first day and can recover from that overnight. If you did muscular work the first day, you may not recover overnight. The only exception is if your aerobic training is trail running and includes running downhill. Then you will want to do your muscular strengthening on the first day after rest and your aerobic the next day.)

- After each strengthening sesssion for your upper body, core, or lower body, allow at least two days off strength training for that part of your body.
- If you strength-train your whole body each time, afterward schedule two rest days from strength training altogether.
- Schedule your light aerobic or flexibility sessions on the same day as you work on strengthening another group of muscles (for example, schedule a brisk walk on the same day you do your upper body strengthening).

IF YOU SCORED 1 OR 2 STARS:

You are very likely a beginner to lifting and muscular strengthening. First and foremost, you need to spend time with your doctor to be sure that there is no pathological problem that is causing your lack of muscular strength or that needs to be treated before you can pursue a strengthening program safely.

If your doctor approves your beginning an exercise program, you need to approach lifting carefully, paying special attention to core strengthening.

As you work your way steadily through your strengthening program, you must give your body the time to adapt to the increasing effort.

Remember, you have the greatest potential to improve.

Weeks 1–3

For the first section of your program, you will want to calendar:

- A one-hour Pilates class or home workout 2 times a week to increase your core strength.
- After each class, when your muscles are warm, spend a half hour doing the following (if you have access to machines):
    - 1 set of 15 to 18 reps of
    - Pull-down/lat machine
    - Horizontal chest press
    - Leg extensions
    - Leg curls
    - Leg press

And with free weights:

- 1 set of 15 to 18 reps of triceps pullover
- 1 set of 15 to 18 reps of biceps curls

If you have no access to weights or weight machines, do 2 sets of push-ups. During each set, perform 50 percent of the repetitions you were able to complete when you tested yourself (for example, if you were able to complete 12 push-ups, perform 2 sets of 6 push-ups each). Rest 2 to 3 minutes between sets. Make sure you maintain good form and a straight back. Exhale when pushing up.

Do some chin-ups. As with push-ups, you can start with 2 sets of 50 percent of the repetitions you can complete in a single series. Rest 2 to 3 minutes between sets. If you cannot perform a chin-up, push yourself up using a chair to support your feet, and hold yourself up for 5 to 8 seconds. Repeat 3 times, with a 1-minute rest in between.

Weeks 4–5

- Continue with 2 one-hour Pilates or core workouts per week.
- Add a second set of 15 to 18 repetitions of both machine and free weights after each class.
- Add a third set of push-ups and chin-ups if you have no access to weight-lifting equipment.

Weeks 6–8

- Continue with 2 one-hour Pilates or core workouts per week.
- Modify the second set by reducing the repetitions to 10 to 12, and increasing the weight to the level that makes your muscles tired for the last 2 repetitions.
- Increase the number of push-ups and chin-ups by 10 to 20 percent.

Weeks 9–12

- Add a third Pilates class or core-strengthening workout.
- Increase your weight lifting by adding a second set of 15 to 18 reps, so

now you should perform 2 sets of 15 to 18 reps and 1 set of 10 to 12 reps for each exercise.

- You can also add 1or 2 more exercises. Since these are going to stress your body through new movements, start with them following the Week 1–3 criteria (1 set of 15 to 18 reps), then progress as you did with the other exercises.

IF YOU SCORED 3 STARS:

Your strength is average. If you have been lifting weights or working on your strength, you can:

Keep doing what you have been doing

or

Step up your level of training, either by increasing the weight you lift or the number of reps you perform

or

Get more sophisticated by alternating 2- to 4-week blocks; one block focusing on muscular endurance, followed by one of strength, and ending with one of power.

If your main activity is aerobic (running, cycling, or Nordic skiing, for example), we suggest you focus on core strengthening. Do Pilates or weight lifting for muscular endurance. You do not want to bulk up because the weight gain—even if from lean mass—could be detrimental to you in your aerobic activity, but you do want to develop muscle that will endure longer against heavier resistance. Some 2- to 3-week blocks to emphasize strength development, if strategically positioned in your plan, can only help. However, limit working on strength when you see a possible negative impact on your technical ability in your specific discipline.

On the other hand, if your main goal is developing muscle size and definition, follow the bodybuilding concept for maximum muscle development by working sets of 8 to 12 reps on isolated muscles following a routine that stresses specific muscle groups in different training sessions. In this case, we counsel you to refer to specific literature or to a good coach.

The following program is designed for the general public, not for those looking to achieve extremes.

Weeks 1–4

For the first section of your program, you will want to calendar:

- A one-hour Pilates or core-strengthening class or home workout 2 times a week.
- After each class, when your muscles are warm, spend 40 to 60 minutes doing 2 sets of 12 to 15 reps of the following upper body exercises. (The following exercise sequence is one possibility. However, you can change exercises/sequence based on your available options.):
- Pull-down lats/lat machine, keeping your hands wider than shoulder width apart, and pulling to your chest, not behind your neck
- Horizontal chest press or bench press with bent knees
- Biceps curls
- Pectoral machine
- One-arm bench row
- Lever or dumbbell lateral raise
- 2 sets of 12 to 15 reps of the following exercises for your lower extremities:
- Leg press or squats using your weight or holding a dumbbell in each hand at a weight that leaves you feeling a little fatigued at the end of 12 to 15 reps. If not, add more. If you have a barbell, do a real squat.
- Leg curls: If you have no access to any equipment, you can use elastic bands. Lie on your stomach with an elastic band (or bike inner tube) around your ankle and anchored to a secure object an adequate distance away. Bring your heel to your glute (butt) by pulling the elastic. You can control the degree of resistance by getting closer or farther from the anchor.
- Leg extensions: These can also be performed without equipment. Just sit on a table that can bear your weight and wrap an elastic band around your ankle. Anchor the elastic to the table leg, and extend your leg against the band's resistance.
- Glutes/hip flexors machine or elastic band.

Weeks 4–5

- Continue with 2 one-hour Pilates or core-strengthening workouts per week.

- Add a third set of 8 to 12 repetitions of both machine and free weights to each exercise.
- Allow a 1- to 2-minute rest between sets.

Weeks 6–8

- Continue with 2 one-hour Pilates or core strengthening workouts per week.
- Modify the second and third sets by reducing the repetitions to 4 to 8 and increasing the weight to the level that makes your muscles tired for the last 2 repetitions.
- Allow a 2- to 3-minute rest between sets.

Weeks 9–12

- In addition to the 2 Pilates or core-strengthening classes with weight lifting afterward, add a third formal lifting session per week. You can also add an extra Pilates class, if your schedule allows. Remember, core strengthening is always a worthwhile investment.
- For these four weeks, we will keep working on strength two times a week and on power once a week. After warming up on a treadmill or cyclette for 10 to 15 minutes, perform a first set of 12 to 15 reps at a comfortable load, followed by 3 to 4 sets of 4 to 6 reps for each exercise. Remember to keep the increased rest of 2 to 3 minutes or more in order to maintain the quality of the effort. You have to feel fatigue when performing the last rep of each set but without losing form.
- For power-training sessions, reduce the weight in order to be able to perform 4 to 5 sets of 6 to 8 reps maintaining the maximum speed of contraction. What's very important at this point is to perform the exercise correctly in order to avoid injury. It's always better to ask someone with more experience to supervise your technique.

IF YOU SCORED 4 STARS:

You already have above-average muscular strength. We normally dedicate the first four weeks of muscular strengthening to muscular adaptation to prepare your body to lift in a safe way. However, if you are already exercising regularly, that may be too easy. Still, we feel that you should dedicate a training block to muscular adaptation anytime you change your lifting routine, you are increasing the amount of lifting, or you are restarting after a period of rest or an injury. In these cases, you always want and need to prepare your muscles for the heavier loads to come in the following weeks. If these first weeks are easy for you, focus on the correct execution of each movement; technical improvements are always a big plus.

Weeks 1–4

- Do at least 8 to 12 exercises:
  divided evenly over your body areas (upper, lower body, midsection)
  or
  dedicated to a specific area if you're training for a specific sport (for example, lower body if you're a skier or a cyclist, upper body if you're a baseball or a tennis player).

- Focus on overall fitness; emphasize midsection exercises.
- Focus on sport-specific exercises.
- Do 3 sets of 12 to 15 repetitions for each exercise.
- Allow 45 seconds to one and a half minutes for recovery between sets.

If you're able to train 3 times a week, train all areas each time. But if you have the option of training 6 times a week, that's ideal. Focus on one area per session and alternate:

- one session for lower body
- one for your core
- one for your upper body and
- repeat

This alternating schedule magnifies the influence the training will have on your muscles.

In general, if you are training for strength, it's better to train one area per session. If you are training for endurance, train all areas.

During this time, you will be targeting skill and adaptation. The more sessions you do, with more rests in between sessions, the more your form will improve.

Week 5

At this point you are probably feeling at home with the proper form for each exercise. Now it's time for you to start working on developing strength.

- For each exercise, perform 1 set of 12 to 15 reps at around 60 percent of your 1RM[1].
- Follow this with 3 sets of 6 to 8 reps using a weight *above* 70 to 75 percent of your 1RM.
- Rest between reps for 1 to 2 minutes.

Weeks 6–7

- After the first set of 12 to 15 reps at 60 percent of 1RM, perform 4 sets of 4 to 5 reps at 90 percent of 1RM (a higher weight than what you had been using earlier in this block), but try to maintain the right form.

Week 8

- After the first set of 12 to 15 reps at 60 percent of 1RM, perform 4 sets of 4 to 5 reps at 70 percent of 1RM (a lower weight than what you had been using earlier in this block), but try to maintain a higher speed of contraction.

Weeks 9–12

Alternate 2 workouts as in the previous block (Weeks 5 and 7) more directed toward developing strength, with one workout dedicated to improving muscular endurance, for example, performing 3 to 4 sets of 15 to 20 reps at 50 percent of 1RM.

Remember, you can use weights in many different combinations of sets, reps, and loads. To keep it simple:

- To develop muscular endurance: Do 3 to 5 sets of 15 to 20 (sometimes more) reps using a weight that is 30 to 50 percent of your 1RM.

---

[1]For information on determining your one repetition maximum, go to page 250.

■ For strength: Do 4 to 6 sets of 2 to 6 reps using the weight that makes the last rep of each set very difficult.

The weight that was 75 to 80 percent of your maximum 12 weeks ago should now be 60 to 70 percent of your max.

IF YOU SCORED 5 STARS:

You are at the top of the chart. Either you picked the right parents or you're already doing the right things. We would like you to not only maintain what you've already achieved but to gain more strength. To do so, continue your current workout at the gym or at home at least 3 to 6 times a week. See if some of our tips can help you. Remember, in most cases to get stronger you have to continue to lift regularly. If you are already feeling you have maximized your lifting, consider changing your routine or your training modality.

Suitable strength-training activities include:

■ machine and free weights
■ Pilates
■ yoga
■ plyometrics
■ rock climbing
■ stair climbing
■ resistance bands
■ surgical tubing
■ stability balls
■ squats
■ toe stands
■ finger walking
■ wall push-ups
■ abdominal crunches
■ biceps curls
■ overhead presses
■ any other exercises that use body weight, such as push-ups and chin-ups

Balance and Coordination

Balance refers to your ability to maintain a position; coordination is your capacity to move through a complex set of movements. These qualities are not fixed, as some believe, but can be vastly improved with use. Improving your balance and coordination enhances the interaction between multiple organs and systems in your body, including your eyes, ears, brain, and nervous system; cardiovascular system; and muscles. Improved balance and coordination can prevent injury, immobility, and many of the aches and pains of daily life. You won't be doing any exercises specifically for balance; you will automatically train your electrical wiring and control tower while doing your aerobic, flexibility, and strength-training activities. However, knowing your starting point and measuring your progress in balance and coordination will be very motivating.

Balance Test

Conduct your test for balance and coordination in a safe area, where you will not get hurt if you lose your balance or fall.

1. Foot-raise: Stand facing a counter, railing or chair about waist high; put your hand on the object for balance. Bend your left knee to bring your left foot off the floor, then drop your hand from the object so you are standing. Time how long you can stand without having to touch anything to keep your balance. If your raised foot touches the floor or you lose your balance, hold on to the object.
2. Repeat with your right foot off the floor, and then again with alternating feet with your eyes closed.

Note the number of seconds you are able to do this without:

- your raised foot touching the support leg
- hopping
- your raised foot touching the floor *or*
- your arms touching something for support

Average your best scores over the four tests. You will be working on balance and coordination in all of the activities that you do. Repeat these balance tests periodically to gauge your improvement.

Six-Week Checkup

The six-week point is the ideal time to retest in order to map your progress. If you try to test earlier than six weeks, your improvement may not be dramatic enough to reveal itself; if you wait longer to test, you may waste additional weeks doing something that's not working for you.

If you score higher than you did on your first test: Your program is working for you. Continue full steam ahead. Do not jump to a higher program.

If you have plateaued (scored the same as you did when you started): Make adjustments to your program using the instructions under Plateaus (see below).

If you scored lower than you had with your first test: Make sure that you are following your exercise prescription precisely. See the instructions, under Fatigue (page 272). But in general:

- be sure that you are allowing for adequate rest
- lighten or eliminate your "active recovery" workout and make it a total rest day
- if you have additional symptoms (a change in eating or sleeping patterns, irritability), see your doctor to find out if you might have an illness (such as an infection, anemia, and so on) that's holding you back

The Art of Adjustments

Along the way, you will need to make adjustments to your schedule. Use the following guidelines to do so effectively.

Plateaus:

If you don't show any further improvement, this is not a sign that the program is wrong for you or you are wrong for exercise. If you already scored 3 to 5 stars, the lack of improvement should merely show that you have already adapted to a great deal of training load and your body no longer perceives these workouts as a stressor. Congratulations! If you only want to retain your current level of fitness, you may continue indefinitely with the schedule you have been using. This level of training is just enough to maintain your level of fitness.

If you scored 1–2 stars at the beginning, followed your program regularly, but you didn't see any improvement, make sure there are no medical reasons that are keeping you from getting better. Also check that your caloric intake is adequate for the increased caloric expenditure that comes with regular training.

If you want to continue to improve:

You now need to modify your program because the one you have been doing doesn't trigger adaptation anymore. Choose one of the following:

1. Change the exercise modality in the area where you have plateaued. For example, if you want to improve your aerobic score, switch to a different aerobic activity, ideally one in which you are not too efficient. If you were walking, start biking; if you were running, swim, do a Spin class, or become a triathlete instead. When you become too good and efficient at one activity, the stress effect on your body can be reduced substantially. This is good when you want to specialize in one discipline, but it requires much more training time for small improvements.

or

2. Increase the volume (number of hours) you train. You can increase 5 to 10 percent every week, for 2- to 4-week cycles, followed by a recovery week in which you reduce your training by 15 percent. You can add a workout every week, or make each workout a little longer. The problem with increasing volume is that time is often a limiting factor, due to work and other commitments.

or

3. Increase the intensity of your training. There are many ways to do so. You can increase the speed or the pace if you are walking or running. You can increase the power if you ride a bike, and you have a power meter. You can go up one notch on the scale of perceived exertion. In strength training, you can increase the amount of weight you're lifting. Another way to increase intensity is to reduce the recovery time between efforts or repetitions (this also saves training time).

or

4. Add competition.

As you reach subsequent plateaus in your new lifelong quest for fitness, choose again from this list to continue to improve.

Fatigue

Some fatigue is normal. Diagnose your fatigue as normal and healthy if you feel good after your rest days or after your easy week. In particular, fatigue shouldn't interfere with your ability to train and perform at your best.

If you are not having days and weeks when you feel good—in other words, if you you always feel fatigued—ask yourself which of the following is most likely true:

- You increased your training load too quickly.
- You are not getting enough recovery time.
- Other stressors in your life may be whittling away at your rest, so you need even more.
- You're not eating enough, particularly carbs; in other words, you increased your exercise load but not your fuel (carbs) intake to the same degree.
- You may have a medical condition, such as anemia, iron deficiency; depression, thyroid dysfunction, or subclinical viral infection.
- You may have overtraining syndrome.

If you increased too quickly: Take a few easy days, then go back to the four-week block that precedes the block when you began to feel fatigue.

If you are not getting enough recovery time: Take two days off after each day or two of training for one or two weeks. To avoid allowing detraining to set in, don't stop completely. Allow more time off in your schedule, then when you start to feel good, increase gradually, only by 5 percent in exercise time every one to two weeks.

If you are not eating enough: See our chapter on nutrition for guidance on the amount of carbohydrates your body needs, particularly before, during, and after exercise.

If you have ruled out the above three, check with your doctor to see if there could be a medical problem impeding your body's ability to recover.

Extreme fatigue

You can also confirm your suspicions of fatigue by measuring your waking heart rate for a few days. When your body experiences very high levels of fatigue, its biological response is a higher resting heart rate. You may find that upon waking your heart rate is 73, well above your normal 58. This means your body is grappling with a very high level of fatigue. If this is the case, you need to continue measuring your resting heart rate to determine when you are physically refreshed enough to start training again. The starting bell dings when your resting heart rate has fallen back to a number that you recognize as normal for you. As you resume exercise, you continue measuring your waking heart rate for one or two days, or if recovering from illness, one week or longer. Once your heart rate is normal, you can resume exercise at full pace.

Unable to finish workouts:

In general, you went too hard or you used an intensity that was too high in relationship to where you are fitnesswise. Go slower or work in a lower training zone for the extent of that workout. For example, if you can't finish the 20-minute workout in Zone 3, go into Zone, 2 until you can finish, then alternate Zones 2 and 3 until you can finish that workout, then increase the time in Zone 3 until you can finish a full workout in Zone 3.

Depression vs. Overtraining:

Fatigue is not always due to something wrong with your training schedule; look at the cumulative stressors in your life. If you feel fatigued when you aren't doing that much exercise, it may be depression. See your doctor and discuss the way you feel. A referral to a sports psychologist or psychiatrist who can administer a Profile of Mood Status or similar tests can be very useful. It's very simple, supplies you with good information, and is much easier than running complex blood workups and other medical tests. If you rule out depression and all potential medical causes of your symptoms, consider overtraining syndrome. Unfortunately, we don't have a biological marker for overtraining, so we first have to exclude medical conditions that can cause a drop in performance (the main element in overtraining syndrome) and fatigue.

Twelve-Week Checkup

Test yourself again. Now continue exercising using the program that applies to your current level of fitness. By now, you should have established a training schedule that works well for you. We hope you have learned enough to be able to manage your training plan by adjusting volume, intensity, modalities, and rest, according to your time availability. We also hope that you feel more in control of your fitness and your health. To accomplish this, pay close attention to your nutritional habits as well.

For the most part, we hope that you have achieved a level of fitness you have never known before, no matter where you started.

> *"Hard* work *pays off in the* future. *Laziness pays off now."*
> —STEVEN WRIGHT, ACADEMY AWARD–WINNING ACTOR
> AND COMEDIAN

faster, better, longer

We want to conclude by sharing with you what folks tell us is very motivating: what you can expect from your new fitness program, the known and not-so-known proven bonuses of fitness. We think it's appropriate to close on this positive note; it also makes it easy for you to open to this information whenever you need inspiration to exercise. Just open to the back of the book and reread a paragraph or two—you'll be back in your gym shoes before you can say "Why be sedentary?"

We've already noted many of the medical bonuses you may experience with exercise. But there are a few more rewards you have to look forward to.

Nature vs. Nurture

We've mentioned that many factors related to your health are genetic, say, about one-tenth to one-quarter. The remaining 75 to 90 percent is due to your habits, and that means that over three-quarters of your total health is influenced by how you live. And as you get older, the power of what you do on a daily basis has even more clout than genetic factors, according to the MacArthur Foundation Study of Successful Aging in America. "If I had known I would live this long, I would've taken better care of myself" could not be more apt. Even low levels of exercise can pack a wallop when it comes to longevity, regardless of genetics. A nineteen-year study performed by the University of Helsinki, Finland, and published in the *Journal of the American*

Medical Association ascertained that among fifteen thousand same-sex twins where one was physically active (defined as exercising at least six times per month, for thirty minutes per session, at the intensity of vigorous walking) and the other twin was sedentary, the twin who exercised had a *55 percent reduced risk of death* compared to the sibling who did not exercise.

According to the *Harvard Medical School Health Letter*, the biological life span of any species is roughly six times the stretch between birth and maturity. Using this formula, the human life span is about 120 years. This is supported by the fact that the human known to have lived the longest so far was a 122-year-old French woman. Within our 120-year life span, however, not only quantity but our quality of life varies enormously. As we said, about one-tenth to one-quarter of that is determined by genes, but the majority of that variance is the result of your lifestyle and environment. That means that you have a tremendous amount of control over how you feel and how long you live. And most of that comes down to how much exercise you have treated your body to. The lifestyle decisions you make every day yield how you will look, feel, move, and even think at forty or eighty.

He Was So Young . . .

"Life is too short to work so hard at it," some say. If you don't, it just might be. Being fit does not simply increase the possibility that you will expand your geriatric years. It also shrinks the chances that you will die during your prime. The British medical journal *Lancet* published the upshot of a twenty-two-year study carried out by a team of Norwegian doctors that showed that even a small increase in fitness significantly lowered the risk of death for people *in their peak productivity years*.

Inactivity Ranks with Smoking

It's hard to believe it now, but there was a time when we didn't actually know that exercise boosted health. In the 1960s and 1970s, scientists and doctors started exploring how disease related to one's negative behavior. In 1961 the Framingham study *proved* that cholesterol correlated with the risk of developing heart disease; a study published in the *British Medical Journal* revealed that lung disease increased in proportion to how much a person smoked. Another study confirmed that drinking alcohol was the single most important cause of liver disease, and so on. Physicians were now able to tell their patients what many docs had suspected for years: The diseases that were killing people were not random, but were linked to negative factors in their lives. Then the scientific community turned its attention to *positive* factors—things you do that positively alter your health. By the mid-nineties, a medical revolution was under way. Scientists and doctors were uncovering a pattern in the conclusions of studies concerning positive factors—namely exercise. By 1996, a U.S. Department of Health and Human Services report detailed that exercise decreases the risk of cardiovascular disease, colon cancer, depression, and noninsulin-dependent diabetes mellitus; that exercise may delay or reduce high blood pressure; and that regular physical activity is necessary for maintaining muscle strength, joint structure, and joint function. The U.S. surgeon general dropped the gavel and judged that inactivity should join its brothers smoking, high blood pressure, and high cholesterol in an infamous league: independent risk factors for a shorter life.

Stronger Longer

Slow suicide. That's what people called smoking back in the seventies, each cigarette one tiny bullet. Now, each day we don't exercise is the current "tiny bullet," a slow kind of suicide.

Not so long ago, staying fit to stave off disease and retain quality of life as humans aged wasn't an issue—we didn't live long enough. Over our millions of years on this planet, our life span has inched up only by tiny increments. In 1900, human life span had only reached forty-seven—just about the age most people now start feeling the pangs of having sat around too much. Since 1900, our life expectancy has shot up dramatically due to disease control. In the last several decades our life span has increased even more markedly. People born in 2000 can expect to live well beyond seventy. But being blessed with such longevity is not all happy times and pass the noisemakers. Indeed, living longer is not always the gift we dream it can be. "Longer life can be a penalty as well as a prize," noted the World Health Organization's *World Health Report* in 1997. "A large part of that price to be paid is in the currency of chronic disease." Medicine, which once struggled with simply keeping people alive, is now grappling with how to help long-living people retain their quality of life. Why? Our well-cushioned lifestyle and technology is catching up with us. Enter: exercise.

I grew up in northern Italy on Lake Como, in a town with steep, winding streets, surrounded by mountains. The town was founded by the Romans many centuries before cars; today traffic is kept outside its medieval walls. I worked there as a family doctor with a practice in the center of town, in a historic building that was the birthplace of the inventor of the battery, Alessandro Volta. Every day I parked outside the city walls and walked or rode a bike to the office, then walked or rode around town to make house calls. The apartment building where I lived outside of town and those I visited on my house calls were all built without elevators. Everyone took the stairs—two, three, four flights each way—and so did I, numerous times a day. Going home in the evening, I felt lucky if I found street parking within a quarter mile of my building. I had no time to exercise regularly, but at age forty-five my weight and cholesterol were perfect.

Then I moved to the U.S. to work at the sports performance clinic in Davis, California, with Eric. In Davis, I drove to the office every day. An elevator in the medical center parking garage delivered me from my car to my desk in a few paces. My patients were just outside the door in the waiting room. In the evening, I marveled that I could pull up, push the electric garage door open, and virtually park in my house.

In twelve months my cholesterol jumped 15 percent and I gained six and a half pounds—and that was with eating more fruits and vegetables, which were abundantly available in California. I had also started going to the gym. However, my level of normal daily activity in Davis still didn't match the level in my previous environment.

People can suffer from high cholesterol for years before displaying any symptoms. Indeed, when I discovered my elevated cholesterol I was surprised. I had been feeling pretty good and thought I was active enough.

For decades I had been touting the medical problems associated with a lifestyle that didn't include movement. Now I was facing it firsthand. The changes in my lifestyle had had an abrupt effect on my body's ability to function well.

—Max

Our early demise is certainly not some sinister plot of our TVs, computers, and cars, but we still cannot ignore the obvious consequences of the machines that now save us from much of the labor-intensive work our body—*every* body—evolved to do. And our bodies are bloating in protest. Many people spend hours every day virtually paralyzed by electronics that require little more activity than the flick of a finger, and their bodies cry out physiologically for action. Hear the cries? Shortness of breath. Aching joints. Sugar, caffeine, and fat mania. Sore backs. Shrinking muscles. XXX-large-sized clothing. Bloating "muffin top" bellies. Cancer. Heart disease. Osteoporosis. Inability to concentrate. Depression. Chronic disease.

Change in Food Supply

Exercise also seems to be the answer to another great modern quandary: food supply. The food supply in the United States morphed in the last hundred years. As recent as the 1970s, one of America's biggest problems was how to feed those who did not have enough to eat. Today, one of our most serious dilemmas is how to help people who have *more* food than they need, and poor-quality food at that. According to data from the Centers for Disease Control and Prevention, in 1991 just four states in the United States had obesity prevalence rates of 15 to 19 percent and no states had rates of 20 percent or above. By 2003, four states had obesity rates above 25 percent, thirty-one states had rates of 20 to 24 percent, and fifteen states had obesity rates of 15 to 19 percent. Over 365,000 people die of obesity-related illnesses in the United States annually—over one thousand human lives lost in the United States every day, many of whom may have been saved if they had gotten the right medicine: exercise. And it impacts youngsters, too. Due to the lack of fitness in today's children, they may be the first generation in the *history of mankind* that will not outlive their parents.

The Fitness Spectrum

Many people believe that the issue of fitness is all or nothing—that you are either fit or nonfit and will eventually get a disease (diabetes, heart attack, stroke) and die. So if you're not dead, you must be fit enough, right? Wrong. It's not just disease that exercise can halt or heal. Aches, reduced function, decreased energy, and other limitations many people struggle with or accept as "aging" are often simply the symptoms of inactivity. Medically speaking, there is a complex gray area between health and disease that is filled with daily complaints: poor digestion, sleep and memory; limited mobility, balance and range of motion; poor eyesight and hearing; fatigue; bad teeth and bad skin; depression, anxiety, and discomfort; bulging midriffs; stiff hands, backs, and gait; and loss of sexual desire and feeling desirable. This isn't death, but is this any kind of a life?

Fitness = Youthfulness

We associate these symptoms with a loss of youth, but a surprising amount of what we think of as "youthfulness" is actually fitness. The surgeon general's report in 1996 pointed up the need for "physical activity for maintaining normal muscle strength, joint structure, and joint function." And, of course, an avalanche of medical literature has been dedicated to the correlation between exercise and weight control, revealing that you not only burn calories while you exercise but you burn more calories 24/7 due to the effect of exercise ratcheting up your resting metabolic rate.

Your Vulnerability to Colds and Flu

Even minor illnesses are beaten back by time on the treadmill. According to the journal *Medicine and Science in Sports and Exercise*, moderately active people showed a 40 percent reduced risk of catching a cold during prime cold season; overall they caught only one upper-respiratory tract infection annually while less active folks suffered through over four. People also experience a reduction in stomach pain, diarrhea, and irritable bowel syndrome when they get some form of physical activity. A study of 1,801 women and men, published in 2005 in *Clinical Gastroenterology and Hepatology*, found obese people who got some form of physical activity were less likely to suffer GI problems than inactive obese people. The study also gleaned that a high Body Mass Index (BMI) was associated with increased symptoms of irritable bowel syndrome, abdominal pain, and diarrhea. Exercise lowers your Body Mass Index.

Your Range of Motion

Exercise improves your ability to perform daily tasks, and your posture and range of motion. Researchers at the University of Florida and the National Institute of Aging working with folks at Stanford University demonstrated that elderly people who elevate their level of regular exercise display superior performance in a test of physical mobility (including balance and speed). They were also less likely to suffer from an age-related disability that hampered their movement. This is good to know, because what do we fear most? Cancer? Death? No, studies reveal that our number-one fear is loss of independence. Exercise may help keep you out of a nursing home.

Meanwhile, it eases back pain and other joint stiffness, including that of your hands, according to researchers at the Mayo Clinic. Finnish researchers added that if you suffer from even very minor stiffness, it may in fact be your body scratching at the door to go for a walk. In a study of eight thousand people they found a correlation between men with arthritis in *one finger* and the risk of heart disease: those with stiffness in one finger were 42 percent likelier to die of heart disease.

The Olympics of Your Daily Life

Exercise also revolutionizes the Olympics of daily life—lifting groceries, doing home improvement projects or hobbies, caring for children or the elderly, gardening, sex. The more strength, power, flexibility, and energy you demand of your body through ever-increasing activity, the more your body will rise to the challenge and grant you the ability to handle that activity. As you exercise, you will get stronger, gain more flexibility, and increase your range of motion, and any given activity in your life will be easier. When you can bench-press two hundred pounds at the gym, you'll find it easier to carry your napping three-year-old son (or grandson). When you're taking yoga classes, putting your hand to the ground is suddenly no big thing—and tying your shoes is a breeze.

Your Eyesight and Hearing

While you're independent and able, you might as well enjoy all the sensory pleasures to the fullest. And exercise helps you do that as well. The Beaver Dam Eye Study, funded by the National Eye Institute, part of the National Institutes of Health, collected information on common eye diseases in six thousand people from age forty-three through eighty-four in Beaver Dam, Wisconsin, not far from Eric's hometown. The investigation concluded that those who were active at least three times a week had *70 percent less chance* of developing age-related macular degeneration. Hearing is not immune to your level of fitness either, according to the *Hearing*

Journal. Researchers behind a study on activity and age-related hearing loss conclude that maintaining a healthy cardiovascular system through regular exercise can lessen the effects of aging on hearing, preventing hearing loss over time.

Your Teeth and Skin

Your teeth will also show gleaming results (unless, Max notes with a smile, you take up boxing). People who are active, eat well, and maintain a normal weight are 40 percent less likely to develop periodontitis, a gum infection that can lead to tooth loss, according to the *Journal of Periodontology*. It has also been shown that gingivitis, which has been linked to heart disease, is improved as well when you take a bite out of inactivity. The *British Journal of Dermatology* released a study whose findings suggest that your skin reflects adaptation to habitual endurance training by increasing its mass and strengthening its structure. That can't hurt the crow's-feet.

If You Need Surgery

Getting in physical shape prior to an operation may also aid in healing. Daniel Rooks, assistant professor of medicine at Harvard Medical School and Beth Israel Deaconess Medical Center in Boston, dissected the disparity among surgical patients who exercised and those who did not, and found that embracing regular exercise prior to having certain surgical procedures has clear benefits, including a speedier recovery.

I have also observed the differences in recovery between people of varying levels of fitness in my surgical practice, in their attitude and in sheer fortitude.

If a patient is interested in returning to their sports, the elite athletes—they *know* they are going to get better, the recreational athlete may, too, but may succumb to the fact that surgery is more than they expected, and the people who aren't fit, well . . .

If you're fit and exposed to surgery, you have a better outcome. It's not that you heal faster or are better at physical therapy, it's that your body can handle the stresses of surgery better. Surgery is very stressful. If you're fit and, say, you can run a marathon, surgery is very similar. If you're fit, surgery is hard on you but your body has the additional resilience and resources to handle it better. If you're not fit, surgery is very, very hard. And sometimes people don't pull through.

—Eric

Your Mood and PMS

The favorable modifying influence of activity on depression has been noted by pretty much everyone: the surgeon general, in conjunction with the U.S. Department of Health and Human Services, CDC, and the National Center for Chronic Disease Prevention and Health Promotion, along with such respected journals as *Psychosomatic Medicine, Archives of the Internal Medicine,* and the *British Journal of Sports Medicine.* A half-dozen "meta-analyses" (studies of studies) have also probed the link between anxiety reduction and exercise, and they observed that the studies agreed unanimously that exercise was significantly related to a reduction in anxiety. A study published in the *British Journal of Clinical Psychology* showed exercise to also profit those with PMS by ameliorating both frequency and severity.

Your Energy Level and Sleep

But you're too tired to work out, you say? Ten minutes of brisk walking can increase your energy levels for up to two hours afterward, note researchers at California State University, Long Beach. Auckland University scientists doubled the stakes, saying that exercise was in fact *better at relieving chronic fatigue than rest.* Regular exercise will also help you get more rest while you sleep. Two different studies (one published in the journal *Sports Medicine* and the other in *Exercise and Sport Science Reviews*) show that exercise significantly increases your total sleep time. More important, when you're active you get more rest from each hour you sleep, because this same research shows that aerobic exercise decreases sleep that includes rapid eye movement (REM). And REM sleep, though deep, does not grant as much rest as sleep that is considered "slow-wave." An inquiry published in the journal *Sleep* awakened the medical community to the fact that both stretching and moderate exercise improved sleep in postmenopausal women, as long as they did not exercise too late in the day. These researchers also spotted that increased fitness with people in general was linked to better sleep.

Your Love Life

It should come as no big surprise that exercise also affects your love life. A Harvard University study of swimmers revealed that regular physical activity correlated with frequency and enjoyment of sexual intercourse. In fact, study participants in their sixties reported sex lives that matched statistics of average forty-year-olds. Research also points up the impact an active lifestyle has on erectile dysfunction, sexual drive, sexual activity, and sexual satisfaction. It's not a reach to imagine that the more time you spend in active pursuits the more often you may find yourself in amorous ones.

Your Mental Acumen

Intellectuals who think exercise is beneath them might want to think again. A group of company executives did, after suffering through protracted negotiations with union truck drivers in the 1960s. When negotiations dragged on, the desk dwellers started making an inordinate number of concessions—because they were getting tired, more tired than the physically fit folks across the negotiating table. Company owners realized that if they were in shape physically, they could sustain their mental sharpness longer at the negotiating table. Better fitness: better concentration.

They weren't the first to catch on to "fit body, fit mind" in action. Astronauts doing mental training also in the 1960s revealed slower response rates the longer the missions ran. An Air Force physician named Dr. Kenneth Cooper made the connection between their waning mental function and their deteriorating physical condition. He surmised that even though the astronauts' tasks were almost entirely mental, their bodies' fatigue due to lack of fitness dampened their brain function.

For the sole purpose of bettering the astronauts' brains, Dr. Cooper put them on a conditioning program that required using large muscle groups in a rhythmic fashion.

Thus, the concept of "aerobics" was born.

More recently the MacArthur Foundation Study of Successful Aging seized upon a similarly astonishing advance: The most physically active seniors were most able to maintain their mental acuity ten years later. Plenty of other animal and human studies have pointed up the relation between exercise and an increase in neural growth factor (NGF), a protein that sets in motion a domino effect in your brain that culminates with even some new brain capillary and neural growth. Sound body, sound mind.

Slow Brain Aging

Not surprising that your brain gets weathered, too, as you age, that your gray matter gets grayer. Your brain makes up only 2 percent of your total body weight (less if you gain weight), yet it gobbles up 20 percent of the energy you consume. The improved circulation of exercise pays dividends to your hungry brain. Building your brain and retaining your neurons also relies on novelty. You are exposed to millions of new bits of sensory "novelty" when you exercise, whether it's on a walk through your neighborhood, a session at the gym or dance studio, or a mountain bike ride up a wilderness trail. Research unearths that the new scenery and faces, the intriguing sounds and sights (particularly the varying light, focal points, and sounds you encounter in the out-of-doors) conspire to bulk up your cognitive skill. Research has found that merely allowing lab rats out of their cages and into the room to explore and exercise, in fact, actually *increases the weight of their brains.*

Work has also been done on the effect of exercise on our youngsters' budding intellects. The *Journal of School Health* published a study that shows that intense physical activity programs have positive effects on academic achievement, including increased concentration; improved mathematics, reading, and writing test scores; and reduced disruptive behavior—even when their activity reduces the time for academics.

Continuing Brain Development

You know you use only a small percentage of your brain. What many don't realize is that what you don't use, you literally lose. You build and reinforce neural connections when you exercise. Think your toddler child or grandchild is building connections when she moves? So are you when you play tag, ball, and Frisbee with her. Research now reveals that this type of brain development continues *throughout adulthood.* And if you were active back when isn't good enough. Your brain is cleansed of unused neurons on a regular basis. With a wide variety of regular activity, you tell your brain you want to hang on to more neurons, including those key neurons in charge of balance, coordination, and muscle movement. Without a variety of physical activity? Down the drain. Whether you're twenty-eight or eighty-eight, you essentially design the brain you want to keep every day through what you do.

A veritable library of research has been cataloged on the correlation of exercise and cognitive function, including some stunning food for thought. A researcher at the Institute for Brain Aging and Dementia at the University of California at Irvine determined that exercise protects animals from developing Alzheimer's-like symptoms. A study published in *Lancet Neurology* reported that people are also less likely to get Alzheimer's if they hit the gym. Exercise also helps you retain what you've already got. A Harvard study also noticed that exercise helped stave off Parkinson's. A British study and the Maastrich Aging Study both recognized that among all age groups (from young folks to those *ninety* and better) those who were more active had speedier information processing. Indulging in new forms of activity in midlife also forces your brain to jump through hoops, creating new synapses.

Does that mean that when you choose the TV over the treadmill today, you may be inadvertently choosing disease tomorrow? When you choose the elevator over the stairs, the lawn service over doing it yourself, a wheelchair? No one can say for certain, but it would be irresponsible for us to say the two are unrelated.

Finally, the Happiness Factor

Despite all of the promise of our fitness program, we don't deny that an important factor for any of us in making a choice is whether or not we think it will make us happy.

It's interesting to note that Harvard psychologist Daniel Gilbert points out that the average person is actually quite *bad* at predicting what will make him happy, and, in fact, Gilbert used exercise to prove it. He did a study in which research subjects strongly believed that a $30,000 increase in income would make them much happier. They felt equally strongly that adding a thirty-minute walk to their daily routine would be of trivial importance. Yet Dr. Gilbert's research suggests that the added income is far less likely to increase happiness than the addition of a regular walk.

So give yourself what is better than a very substantial raise. You have a lot to look forward to. Go to it. We'll keep you updated with new research and exercise information at www.fasterbetterstronger.com. And send us an e-mail—we'd love to hear how exercise has improved your life.

endnotes

Here we detail the most relevant studies that we reference throughout the book. We all owe a great debt of gratitude to these scientists who have scrupulously researched and uncovered these facts; they are the true pioneers in bringing exercise home to all of us. Rather than footnoting, we index these studies by subject for your easy reference or if you would like to investigate a topic further. In addition, we have included the study of summaries where possible, which makes for very interesting and informative reading.

Cholesterol and Heart Disease

Kannel, W.B., Dawber, T.R., Kagan, A., Revotskie, N., Stokes, J., 3rd. Factors of risk in the development of coronary heart disease—six-year follow-up experience. The Framingham Study. *Annals of Internal Medicine* 1961; 55:33–50.

The Framingham study established a relationship between the levels of cholesterol and risk for cardiovascular disease. Further, the study established a strong positive association of LDL cholesterol with coronary heart disease as well as a powerful inverse and protective effect of HDL levels.

Smoking and Lung Disease

Doll, R., Hill, A.B. Smoking and carcinoma of the lung. Preliminary report. *British Medical Journal* 2 1950 Sep 30; 4682:739–748.

The risk of developing [lung] disease increases in proportion to the amount smoked. It may be fifty times as great among those who smoke twenty-five or more cigarettes a day as among nonsmokers.

Alcohol and Liver Disease

Grant, B.F., Dufour, M.C., and Harford, T.C. Epidemiology of alcoholic liver disease. *Seminars in Liver Disease* 1988; 8(1):12–25.

Chronic excessive alcohol use is the single most important cause of illness and death from liver disease (alcoholic hepatitis and cirrhosis) in the United States.

U.S. Surgeon General and Lack of Exercise

U.S. Department of Health and Human Services. *Physical Activity and Health: A Report of the Surgeon General.* Atlanta, Georgia: U.S. Department of Health and Human Services, Centers for Disease Control and Prevention, National Center for Chronic Disease Prevention and Health Promotion,1996.

Physical Activity and Health: A Report of the Surgeon General is a comprehensive overview of research related to physical activity and health. The report (1) summarizes the benefits of physical activity, (2) reinforces the importance of promoting physical activity, (3) states that many children and adolescents are at risk for health problems because of inactive lifestyles, and (4) states that everyone should participate in a moderate amount of physical activity (fifteen minutes of running, thirty minutes of brisk walking, forty-five minutes of playing volleyball) on most, if not all, days of the week.

Exercise and Coronary Artery Disease

U.S. Department of Health and Human Services. *Physical Activity and Health: A Report of the Surgeon General.* Atlanta, GA: U.S. Department of Health and Human Services, Centers for Disease Control and Prevention, National Center for Chronic Disease Prevention and Health Promotion,1996. http://www.cdc.gov/nccdphp/sgr/sgr.htm

Regular physical activity or cardiorespiratory fitness decreases the risk of cardiovascular disease mortality in general and of coronary heart disease mortality in particular.

Kraus, W.E., Houmard, J.A., Duscha, B.D., Knetzger, K.J., Wharton, M.B., McCartney, J.S., Bales, C.W., Henes, S., Samsa, G.P., Otvos, J.D., Kulkarni, K.R., Slentz, C.A. Effects of the amount and intensity of exercise on plasma lipoproteins. *New England Journal of Medicine* 2002 Nov 7; 347 (19):1483–1492.

Increased physical activity is related to reduced risk of cardiovascular disease, possibly because it leads to improvement in the lipoprotein profile.

Exercise and Cerebrovascular Disease (Stroke)

Gorelick, P.B., Sacco, R.L., Smith, D.B., Alberts, M., Mustone-Alexander, L., Rader, D. et al. Prevention of a first stroke: a review of guidelines and a multidisciplinary consensus statement from the National Stroke Association. *The Journal of the American Medical Association* 1999 Mar 24/31; 281:1112–1120.

Physical activity may help prevent stroke. The Prevention Advisory Board of the National Stroke Association (NSA) recommends taking "a brisk walk for as little as thirty minutes a day" as one of ten strategies to help prevent stroke, America's leading cause of adult disability. Regular exercise may help prevent strokes, the recommendations note, in part because physical activity positively affects many risk factors. Physical activity can help control blood pressure and that's the leading risk factor for stroke.

Exercise and Hypertension

U.S. Department of Health and Human Services. *Physical Activity and Health: A Report of the Surgeon General*. Atlanta, GA: U.S. Department of Health and Human Services, Centers for Disease Control and Prevention, National Center for Chronic Disease Prevention and Health Promotion,1996. http://www.cdc.gov/nccdphp/sgr/sgr.htm

Regular physical activity prevents or delays the development of high blood pressure, and exercise reduces blood pressure in people with hypertension.

American Heart Association. *2002 Heart and Stroke Statistical Update*. Dallas: American Heart Association, 2001. 23–24.

Regular exercise can lower your blood pressure. Less active, less fit persons have a 30 to 50 percent greater risk of developing high blood pressure.

Blumenthal, J.A., Sherwood, A., Gullette, E.C.D., Babyak, M.A., Waugh, R., Georgiades, A., Craidhead, L.W., Tweedy, D., Feinglos, M., Appelbaum, M., Hayano, J., Hinderliter, A. Exercise and weight loss reduce blood pressure in men and women with mild hypertension. *Archives of Internal Medicine* 2000 July; 160(13):1947–1958.

Although exercise alone was effective in reducing BP, the addition of a behavioral weight-loss program enhanced this effect. Aerobic exercise combined with weight loss is recommended for the management of elevated BP in sedentary, overweight individuals.

Exercise and Diabetes

U.S. Department of Health and Human Services. *Physical Activity and Health: A Report of the Surgeon General*. Atlanta, GA: U.S. Department of Health and Human Services, Centers for Disease Control and Prevention, National Center for Chronic Disease Prevention and Health Promotion,1996. http://www.cdc.gov/nccdphp/sgr/sgr.htm

Regular physical activity lowers the risk of developing non-insulin-dependent diabetes mellitus.

Wing, R. et al. (Diabetes Prevention Program Research Group). Reduction in the incidence of type 2 diabetes with lifestyle intervention or metformin. *New England Journal of Medicine* 2002 Feb 7; 346:393–403.

Millions of overweight Americans at high risk for type 2 diabetes can delay and possibly prevent the disease with moderate diet and exercise. Lifestyle changes and treatment with metformin both reduced the incidence of diabetes in persons at high risk. The lifestyle intervention was more effective than metformin.

Gregg, E.W., Gerzoff, R.B., Caspersen, C.J. et al. Relationship of walking to mortality among U.S. adults with diabetes. *Archives of Internal Medicine* 2003;163:1440–1447.

Demonstrated that [walking] substantially reduces the chances of developing diabetes.

Exercise and Excess Weight

Jakicic, J.M., Marcus, B.H., Gallagher, K.I., Napolitano, M., Lang, W. Effect of exercise duration and intensity on weight loss in overweight, sedentary women: a randomized trial. *Journal of the American Medical Association* 2003; 290:1323–1330.

If you are exercising mainly to lose weight or maintain a healthy weight, thirty minutes or so a day will work if you're careful about how much you eat.

Ballor, D., Poehlman, E. Resting metabolic rate and coronary heart risk in aerobically and resistance trained women. *American Journal of Clinical Nutrition* 1992; 56:968–1974.

Broeder, C., Burrhus, K. et al. The effects of either high intensity resistance or endurance training on resting metabolic rate. *American Journal of Clinical Nutrition* 1992; 55:802–810.

Campbell, W., Crim, M. et al. Increased energy requirements and changes in body composition with resistance training in older adults. *American Journal of Clinical* Nutrition 1994; 60:167–175.

[These three] studies have shown strength training to increase lean body mass, decrease fat mass, and increase resting metabolic rate (a measurement of the amount of calories burned per day). These effects may make it easier to manage one's weight.

Exercise and Obesity

Miller, W.C., Koceja, D.M., Hamilton, E.J. A meta-analysis of the past twenty-five years of weight loss research using diet, exercise, or diet plus exercise intervention. *International Journal of Obesity* 1997 Oct; 21(10):941–947.

The data shows that a fifteen-week diet, or diet plus exercise program, produces a weight loss of about 11 kg, with a 6.6±0.5 and 8.6±0.8 kg maintained loss after one year, respectively.

You, T., Murphy, K.M., Lyles, M.F., Demons, J.L., Lenchik, L., Nicklas, B.J. Addition of aerobic exercise to dietary weight loss preferentially reduces abdominal adipocyte size. *International Journal of Obesity* 2006; 30:1211–1216.

Addition of exercise training to dietary weight loss preferentially reduces subcutaneous abdominal adipocyte size in obese women.

Exercise and Cholesterol

Varady, K.A., Jones, P.J.H. The American Society for Nutritional Sciences. Combination diet and exercise interventions for the treatment of dyslipidemia: an effective preliminary strategy to lower cholesterol levels? *Journal of Nutrition* 2005 Aug; 135:1829–1835.

These findings suggest that combination lifestyle therapies are an efficacious, preliminary means of improving cholesterol levels in those diagnosed with dyslipidemia, and should be implemented in place of drug therapy when cholesterol levels fall just above the normal range.

Exercise and Musculoskeletal Diseases

U.S. Department of Health and Human Services. *Physical Activity and Health: A Report of the Surgeon General.* Atlanta, GA: U.S. Department of Health and Human Services, Centers for Disease Control and Prevention, National Center for Chronic Disease Prevention and Health Promotion, 1996. http://www.cdc.gov/nccdphp/sgr/sgr.htm

Regular physical activity is necessary for maintaining normal muscle strength, joint structure, and joint function. In the range recommended for health, physical activity is not associated with joint damage or development of osteoarthritis and may be beneficial for many people with arthritis. Weight-bearing physical activity is essential for normal skeletal development during childhood and adolescence and for achieving and maintaining peak bone mass in young adults.

Exercise and Bone Density

Nelson, M.E., Fiatarone, C.M. et al. Effects of high-intensity strength training on multiple risk factors for osteoporotic fractures. A randomized controlled trial. *Journal of the American Medical Association* 1994; 272:1909–1914.

Another beneficial effect of resistance training pertains to bone health. In addition to weight-bearing cardiovascular exercise, weight training has been shown to help fight osteoporosis. For example, in postmenopausal women, two strength training sessions a week for one year increased bone mineral density by 1 percent. A sedentary control group lost 2 percent in the same time period.

Exercise and Joint ROM/Degenerative Arthritis

Ettinger, Jr., W.H. et al. A randomized trial comparing aerobic exercise and resistance exercise with a health education program in older adults with knee osteoarthritis the fitness arthritis and seniors trial (FAST). *Journal of the American Medical Association* 1997; 277:25–31.

Participation in regular exercise appears to be safe and effective in managing the symptoms and disability associated with osteoarthritis.

Kovar, P.A. et al. Supervised fitness walking in patients with osteoarthritis of the knee. A randomized, controlled trial. *Annals of Internal Medicine* 1992; 116:529–534.

A program of supervised fitness walking and

patient education can improve functional status without worsening pain or exacerbating arthritis-related symptoms in patients with osteoarthritis of the knee.

Exercise and Cancer

Fleeger, Fran, M.D., Berman, John, Hanc, John. *The Force Program*. New York: Ballantine Books, 2001.

The Force Program works with traditional cancer treatments to speed recovery and prevent recurrence. Designed for easy at-home use, step-by-step exercises are tailored to the needs and abilities of all patients, from bedridden nonathletes to trained competitors. Nutritional advice helps maximize the body's ability to fight cancer. A complete guide to stress management helps improve responses to pain, tension, and upsetting situations.

Exercise and Cancer: Colon

U.S. Department of Health and Human Services. *Physical Activity and Health: A Report of the Surgeon General*. Atlanta, GA: U.S. Department of Health and Human Services, Centers for Disease Control and Prevention, National Center for Chronic Disease Prevention and Health Promotion,1996. http://www.cdc .gov/nccdphp/sgr/sgr.htm

Regular physical activity is associated with a decreased risk of colon cancer.

Simon, Harvey B. Can you run away from cancer? Harvard Health Letter Mar 1992.

"Since 1980 at least eight studies have examined the relationship between physical activity and colon cancer; seven have concluded that exercise reduces the risk."

McTiernan, A. et al. Effect of a 12-month exercise intervention on patterns of cellular proliferation in colonic crypts: a randomized controlled trial. *Cancer Epidemiology, Biomarkers and Prevention* Sep 2006; 15:1588–1597.

Aerobic exercise may play a major role in reducing the risk of colon cancer and colon polyps in men.

Exercise and Cancer: Breast

McTiernan, A., Kooperberg, C., White, E. et al. Recreational physical activity and the risk of breast cancer in postmenopausal women: the Women's Health Initiative cohort study. *Journal of the American Medical Association* 2003; 290:1331–1336.

Physical activity significantly reduced the risk of breast cancer in postmenopausal women, whether the activity was strenuous or not.

Rose, E. Frisch et al. Lower prevalence of breast cancer and cancers of the reproductive system among former college athletes compared to nonathletes. *British Journal of Cancer* 1985; 52(6):885–891.

The best study of exercise and breast cancer . . . evaluated the lifetime risk of breast cancer in 5,398 alumnae of ten colleges and universities. Researchers grouped the women according to their participation in college sports and assumed that former athletes would be more active than nonathletes throughout life. The differences between the two groups were striking: nonathletes had 86 percent more breast cancer than the team players.

King, M.C., Marks, J.H., Mandell, J.B. Breast and ovarian cancer risks due to inherited mutations in BRCA1 and BRCA2. *Science* 2003; 302:643–645.

Physical exercise and lack of obesity in adolescence were associated with significantly delayed breast cancer onset.

Exercise and Cancer: Prostate

Barnard, R.J. et al. Effect of diet and exercise on serum insulin, IGF-I, and IGFBP-1 levels and growth of LNCaP cells in vitro. *Cancer Causes and Control* 2002; 13(10):929–935.

UCLA scientists report that eleven days of daily exercise and the Pritikin low-fat, high-fiber diet induce prostate cancer cells to die. The research is the first to show that diet and exercise can kill prostate cancer cells.

Giovannucci, E. et al. A prospective study of physical activity and incident and fatal prostate cancer. *Archives of Internal Medicine* 2005 May 9; 165:1005–1010.

Older men who exercise regularly have a much lower risk of dying from prostate cancer. The study showed that men over age sixty-five who engaged in at least three hours of vigorous physical activity, such as running, biking, or swimming, per week had a nearly 70 percent lower risk of being diagnosed with advanced prostate cancer or dying from the disease.

Exercise and COPD (Chronic Obstructive Pulmonary Disease)

Casaburi, R., Patessio, A., Ioli, F. et al. Reductions in exercise lactic acidosis and ventilation as a result of exercise training in patients with obstructive lung disease. *American Review of Respiratory Disease* 1991; 143:9–18.

Patients with moderate chronic obstructive pulmonary disease (COPD) derive a greater physiological training benefit if exercise is performed at a work rate that exceeds their anaerobic threshold.

Emery, Charles et al. Acute effects of exercise on cognition in patients with chronic obstructive pulmonary disease. *American Journal of Respiratory and Critical Care Medicine* 2001 Nov; 164(9):1624–1627.

A new study suggests that a single, short burst of moderately intense exercise gives a mental boost to people with a serious lung disease. Immediately after twenty minutes of riding a stationary bicycle, people with chronic obstructive pulmonary disease (COPD) showed improvement in cognitive function.

Emery, C.F., Schein, R.L., Hauck, E.R., MacIntyre, N.R. Psychological and cognitive outcomes of a randomized trial of exercise among patients with chronic obstructive pulmonary disease. *Health Psychology* 1998 May; 17(3):232–240.

Regular exercise can help people with serious lung disease reduce anxiety and depression and improve endurance and some kinds of intellectual functioning, a new study shows. This research was the first randomized study to find specifically that exercise can reduce anxiety for patients with chronic obstructive pulmonary disease (COPD).

Exercise and Depression

U.S. Department of Health and Human Services. *Physical Activity and Health: A Report of the Surgeon General.* Atlanta, GA: U.S. Department of Health and Human Services, Centers for Disease Control and Prevention, National Center for Chronic Disease Prevention and Health Promotion,1996. http://www.cdc.gov/nccdphp/sgr/sgr.htm

Physical activity appears to relieve symptoms of depression and anxiety and improve mood. Regular physical activity may reduce the risk of developing depression, although further research is required on this topic.

Babyak, M., Blumenthal, J.A., Herman, S., Khatri, P., Doraiswamy, P.M., Moore, K., Craighead, W.E., Baldewicz, T.T., and Krishnan, K.R. Exercise treatment for major depression: maintenance of therapeutic benefit at 10 months. *Psychosomatic Medicine* 2000 Sept/Oct; 62:633–638.

Findings suggest that a modest exercise program is an effective, robust treatment for patients with major depression who are positively inclined to participate in it. The benefits of exercise are likely to endure particularly among those who adopt it as a regular, ongoing life activity.

Blumenthal, J.A., Babyak, M.A., Moore, K.A., Craighead, W.E., Herman, S., Khatri, P., Waugh, R., Napolitano, M.A., Forman, L.M., Appelbaum, M., Doraiswamy, P.M., Krishnan, K.R. Effects of exercise training on older patients with major depression. *Archives of Internal Medicine* 1999 Oct 25; 159:2349–2356.

An exercise training program may be considered an alternative to antidepressants for treatment of depression in older persons. Although antidepressants may facilitate a more rapid initial therapeutic response than exercise, after sixteen weeks of treatment, exercise was equally effective in reducing depression among patients with MDD.

Dimeo, F., Bauer, M., Varahram, I., Proest, G., Halter, U. Benefits from aerobic exercise in patients with major depression: a pilot study. *British Journal of Sports Medicine* 2001 Apr; 35(2):114–117.

Aerobic exercise can produce substantial improvement in mood in patients with major depressive disorders in a short time.

Exercise and PMS

Aganoff, J.A. et al. Aerobic exercise, mood states and menstrual cycle symptoms. *Journal of Psychosomatic Research* 1994 Apr; 38(3):183–192.

Steege, J.F. et al. The effects of aerobic exercise on premenstrual symptoms in middle-aged women: a preliminary study. Journal of Psychosomatic Research 1993; 37(2):127–133.

Choi, P.Y. et al. Symptom changes across the menstrual cycle in competitive sportswomen, exercisers and sedentary women. *British Journal of Clinical Psychology* 1995; 34(3):447–460.

Summary of three studies combined: Exercise has a favorable modifying influence on PMS frequency and severity. Several studies demonstrate that women who engage in regular exercise programs do not suffer from PMS nearly as often as sedentary women. In addition to lowering free-estrogen blood levels, exercise also raises brain endorphin levels, improving mood and reducing anxiety and feelings of depression.

Exercise and Colds and Flu

Matthews, C.E. et. al. Moderate to vigorous physical activity and risk of upper respiratory tract infection. *Medicine and Science in Sports and Exercise* 2002;

34(8):1242–1248. Findings showed that the group who got at least moderate exercise on most days averaged one cold, while the less active group reported over four colds in the year. The most obvious benefit to exercise appeared in the fall when nearly 40 percent of the colds were reported. The active group showed a risk reduction of 32 percent during the prime season for colds.

Ulrich, C.M. et. al. Fred Hutchinson Cancer Research Center. Moderate-intensity exercise reduces the incidence of colds among postmenopausal women. *The American Journal of Medicine* 2006 Nov; 119:11.

A moderate exercise program may reduce the incidence of colds. The trial is the first to report on the effects of a year-long, moderate-intensity exercise training program on the incidence of upper respiratory tract infections. Although we did not find an effect overall on upper respiratory tract infections, our study suggests that moderate-intensity training can reduce the risk of colds in postmenopausal, nonsmoking, overweight, or obese women. This finding is of clinical relevance and adds a new facet to the growing literature on the health benefits of moderate exercise.

Exercise and the Release of Endorphins

Taylor, D.V., Boyajian, J.G., James, N., Woods, D., Chicz-Demet, A., Wilson, A.F., Sandman, C.A. Acidosis stimulates beta-endorphin release during exercise. *Journal of Applied Physiology* 1994; 77(4): 1913–1918.

Exercise-induced acidosis of the blood appears when prolonged exercise has occurred and oxygen flow to the muscles has decreased. Anaerobic respiration occurs causing lactic acid accumulation, which results in acidosis. This acidosis is then thought to stimulate the pituitary to release the endorphins.

Exercise and Resting Metabolic Rate

Ballor, D., Poehlman, E. Resting metabolic rate and coronary heart risk in aerobically and resistance trained women. *American Journal of Clinical Nutrition* 1992; 56:968–974.

Broeder, C., Burrhus, K. et al. The effects of either high intensity resistance or endurance training on resting metabolic rate. *American Journal of Clinical Nutrition* 1992; 55:802–810.

Campbell, W., Crim, M. et al. Increased energy requirements and changes in body composition with resistance training in older adults. *American Journal of Clinical Nutrition* 1994; 60:167–175.

These three studies have shown strength training to increase lean body mass, decrease fat mass, and increase resting metabolic rate (a measurement of the amount of calories burned per day). These effects may make it easier to manage one's weight.

Borsheim, E., Bahr, R. Effect of exercise intensity, duration and mode on post-exercise oxygen consumption. *Sports Medicine* 2003; 33(14):1037–1060.

The exercise after-burn, or the calories expended (above resting values) after an exercise bout, is referred to as "excess post-exercise oxygen consumption," or EPOC. This represents the oxygen consumption above resting level that the body is utilizing to return itself to its pre-exercise state. The physiological mechanisms responsible for this increased metabolism (all chemical reactions in the body to liberate energy that is measured by oxygen consumption) include the replenishment of oxygen stores, phosphagen (ATP-PC) resynthesis, lactate removal, and the increased ventilation, blood circulation, and body temperature above pre-exercise levels.

Exercise and Sleep

Tworoger, S.S., Yasui, Y., Vitiello, M.V. et al. Effects of a yearlong moderate-intensity exercise and a stretching intervention on sleep quality in postmenopausal women. *Sleep* 2003; 26(7):830–836.

Both stretching and exercise interventions may improve sleep quality in sedentary, overweight, postmenopausal women. Increased fitness was associated with improvements in sleep. However, the effect of moderate-intensity exercise may depend on the amount of exercise and time of day it is performed.

Kubitz, K.K., Landers, D.M., Petruzzello, S.J., Han, M.W. The effects of acute and chronic exercise on sleep. *Sports Medicine* 1996; 21(4), 277–291.

O'Connor, P.J., Youngstedt, M.A. Influence of exercise on human sleep. Exercise and Sport Science Reviews 1995; 23:105–134.

Both studies show that exercise significantly increases total sleep time and aerobic exercise decreases rapid eye movement (REM) sleep. REM sleep is a paradoxical form in that it is a deep sleep, but it is not as restful as slow wave sleep.

Lamprecht, S.A., Lipkin, M. Chemoprevention of colon cancer by calcium, vitamin D and folate: molecular mechanisms. *Nature Reviews Cancer* 2003; 3:601–614.

Van den Bemd, G.J., Chang, G.T. Vitamin D and vitamin D analogs in cancer treatment. *Current Drug Targets* 2002; 3:85–94.

The above two studies show vitamin D reduces the risk of cancer. Reasons include enhancing calcium absorption (in the case of colorectal cancer) (Lamprecht and Lipkin, 2003), inducing cell differentiation, increasing cancer cell apoptosis or death, reducing metastasis and proliferation, and reducing angiogenesis.

Exercise and Decreased Anxiety

Calfas, K.J., Taylor, W.C. Effects of physical activity on psychological variables in adolescents. *Pediatric Exercise Science* 1994; 6:406–423.

Kugler, J., Seelback, H., Krüskemper, G.M. Effects of rehabilitation exercise programmes on anxiety and depression in coronary patients: A meta-analysis. *British Journal of Clinical Psychology* 1994; 33:401–410.

Landers, D.M., Petruzzello, S.J. Physical activity, fitness, and anxiety. In C. Bouchard, R.J. Shephard, and T. Stevens (eds.). *Physical activity, fitness, and health.* Champaign, IL: Human Kinetics Publishers, 1994.

Long, B.C., van Stavel, R. Effects of exercise training on anxiety: A meta-analysis. *Journal of Applied Sport Psychology* 1995; 7:167–189.

McDonald, D.G., Hodgdon, J.A. *The psychological effects of aerobic fitness training: Research and theory.* New York: Springer-Verlag, 1991.

Petruzzello, S.J., Landers, D.M., Hatfield, B.D., Kubitz, K.A., Salazar, W. A meta-analysis on the anxiety-reducing effects of acute and chronic exercise. *Sports Medicine* 1991; 11(3):143–182.

There have been six meta-analyses examining the relationship between exercise and anxiety reduction. All six of these meta-analyses found that across all studies examined, exercise was significantly related to a reduction in anxiety. These effects ranged from "small" to "moderate" in size and were consistent for trait, state, and psychophysiological measures of anxiety.

Hassmen, P., Koivula, N., Uutela, A. Physical exercise and psychological well-being: a population study in Finland. *Preventive Medicine* 2000 Jan; 30(1):17–25. The results of this cross-sectional study suggest that individuals who exercised at least two

to three times a week experienced significantly less depression, anger, cynical distrust, and stress than those exercising less frequently or not at all. Furthermore, regular exercisers perceived their health and fitness to be better than less frequent exercisers did.

Exercise and Self-Esteem

Calfas, K.J., Taylor, W.C. Effects of physical activity on psychological variables in adolescents. *Pediatric Exercise Science* 1994; 6:406–423.

Gruber, J.J. Physical activity and self-esteem development in children. *Effects of physical activity and self-esteem development in children.* Champaign, IL: Human Kinetics Publishers,1986.

McDonald, D.G., Hodgdon, J.A. *The psychological effects of aerobic fitness training: Research and theory.* New York: Springer-Verlag, 1991.

Spence, J.C., Poon, P., Dyck, P. The effect of physical-activity participation on self-concept: a meta-analysis. *Journal of Sport and Exercise Psychology* 1997; 19:109.

All four of the reviews found that physical activity/exercise brought about small, but statistically significant, increases in physical self-concept or self-esteem. These effects generalized across gender and age groups.

Exercise and Eyesight

Knudtson, M.D. et al. Physical activity and the 15-year cumulative incidence of age-related macular degeneration: the Beaver Dam Eye Study. *British Journal of Ophthalmology* 2006 Oct 31; 2006; 0:1–3.

Older individuals who stay active and exercise for at least three times a week have 70 percent less chance of developing age-related macular degeneration.

Exercise and Longevity

Lee, I.M., Hsieh, C.C., Paffenbarger, R.S. Exercise intensity and longevity in men. *The Journal of the American Medical Association* 1995 Apr 19; 273(15):1179–1184.

The study has clearly demonstrated that exercise is associated with a lower death rate. Furthermore, the more you exercise, the greater the benefit.

Sherman, S.E. et al. Physical activity and mortality in women in the Framingham Heart Study. *American Heart Journal* 1994 Nov; 128(5):879–884.

Dr. Sherman reported on 1,404 women aged fifty

to seventy-four who were free of cardiovascular disease. The most active group had a 33 percent lower death rate than the least active. Therefore, it was concluded that women who were more active lived longer.

Lissner, L. et al. Physical activity levels and changes in relation to longevity. A prospective study of Swedish women. *American Journal of Epidemiology* 1996 Jan 1; 143(1):54–62.

Another study of Swedish women demonstrated that mortality was dramatically reduced in women who had physically active jobs or who frequently participated in a leisure-time activity. It was concluded that decreases in physical activity, as well as low initial levels of activity, are strong risk factors for mortality in women, and that their predictive values persist for many years.

Franco, Oscar H., M.D., Ph.D. et al. Effects of Physical Activity on Life Expectancy with Cardiovascular Disease. *Archives of Internal Medicine* Nov 2005; 165(20):2355–2360.

The researchers looked at records of more than five thousand middle-aged and elderly Americans and found that those who had moderate to high levels of activity lived 1.3 to 3.7 years longer than those who got little exercise, largely because they put off developing heart disease—the nation's leading killer. Men and women benefited about equally.

Exercise and Sex

Krucoff, C., Krucoff, M. Peak performance. *American Fitness* 2000; 19:32–36.

A Harvard University study of 160 male and female swimmers in their forties and sixties showed a positive relationship between regular physical activity and the frequency and enjoyment of sexual intercourse. Results stated swimmers in their sixties reported sex lives comparable to people in the general population in their forties.

Bortz, W. M., Wallace, D.H. Physical fitness, aging, and sexuality. *Western Journal of Medicine* 1999; 170:167–175.

A high level of sexual activity and satisfaction to be correlated with degree of fitness in both older men and women.

Stanten, N., Yeager S. Four workouts to improve your love life. *Prevention* 2003; 55:76–78.

Research indicates that exercise may increase sexual drive, sexual activity, and sexual satisfaction. Results of a recent study reported that women were more sexually responsive following twenty minutes of vigorous exercise.

Esposito, K. et. al. Effect of lifestyle changes on erectile dysfunction in obese men. *Journal of the American Medical Association* 2004 June 23/30; 291:2978–2984.

In our study, about one-third of obese men with erectile dysfunction regained their sexual function after two years of adopting healthy behaviors, mainly regular exercise and reducing weight.

Bacon, C. et al. Sexual function in men older than 50 years of age. *Annals of Internal Medicine* 2003 Aug 5; 139:161–168.

After studying some 31,000 men between ages fifty-five and ninety, the researchers show that men who regularly exercised typically had a ten-year delay in erectile dysfunction compared with more sedentary guys.

Exercise and Increased Improvement with Age

Woo, J.S., Derleth, C., Stratton, J.R., Levy, W.C. The influence of age, gender, and training on exercise efficiency. *Journal of the American College of Cardiology* 2006; 47:1049–1057.

Exercise and POMS

Terry, P.C., Lane, A.M., Lane, H.J., Keohane, L. Development and validation of a mood measure for adolescents. *Journal of Sports Sciences* 1999; 17: 861–872.

The aim of this study was to develop and validate a shortened version of the Profile of Mood States suitable for use with adolescents.

McNair, D., Lorr, M., Droppleman, L. *Manual for the Profile of Mood States.* San Diego, CA: Educational and Industrial Testing Service, 1971.

Morgan, W.P. Test of champions: The iceberg profile. *Psychology Today* 1980; 14:92–99, 102, 108.

Exercise and Our Brain

Blumenthal, J. et al. Effects of exercise training on cognitive functioning among depressed older men and women. *Journal of Aging and Physical Activity* 2001 Jan; 9(1).

Aerobic exercise in middle-aged and elderly patients improved their cognitive abilities.

The researchers found significant improvements in the higher mental processes of memory and the so-called executive functions, which include planning, organization, and the ability to mentally juggle different intellectual tasks at the same time.

Barnes, D.E., Yaffe, K., Satariano, W.A., Tager, I.B. A longitudinal study of cardiorespiratory fitness and cognitive function in healthy older adults. *Journal of the American Geriatrics Society* 2003 Apr; 51:459–465.

Baseline measures of cardiorespiratory fitness are positively associated with preservation of cognitive function over a six-year period and with levels of performance on cognitive tests conducted six years later in healthy older adults. High cardiorespiratory fitness may protect against cognitive dysfunction in older people.

Abbott, R.D., White, L.R., Ross, G.W., Masaki, K.H., Curb, D., Petrovitch, H. Walking and dementia in physically capable elderly men. *Journal of the American Medical Association* 2004 Sept 22; 292:1447–1453.

The researchers concluded that their findings "suggest that walking is associated with a reduced risk of dementia" and that "promoting active lifestyles in physically capable men could help late-life cognitive function."

Weuve, J., Kang, J.H., Manson, J.E., Breteler, M.M.B., Ware, J.H., Grodstein, F. Physical activity, including walking, and cognitive function in older women. *Journal of the American Medical Association* 2004 Sept 22; 292:454–1461.

Long-term regular physical activity, including walking, is associated with significantly better cognitive function and less cognitive decline in older women.

Symons, C.W., Cinelli, B., James, T.C., Groff, P. Bridging student health risks and academic achievement through comprehensive school health programs. *Journal of School Health* 1997; 67(6): 220–227.

Intense physical activity programs have positive effects on academic achievement, including increased concentration; improved mathematics, reading, and writing test scores; and reduced disruptive behavior. Academic achievement improves even when the physical education reduces the time for academics.

Adlard, P.A., Cotman, C.W. et al. Voluntary exercise decreases amyloid load in a transgenic model of Alzheimer's disease. *Journal of Neuroscience* 2005 Apr 27; 25:4217–4221.

Long-term physical activity enhances the learning ability of mice and decreases the level of plaque-forming beta-amyloid protein fragments—a hallmark characteristic of Alzheimer's disease (AD)—in their brains.

Rovio, S., Kåreholt, I., Helkala, E.L., Viitanen, M., Winblad, B., Tuomilehto, J., Soininen, H., Nissinen, A., Kivipelto, M. Leisure-time physical activity at midlife and the risk of dementia and Alzheimer's disease. *Lancet Neurology* 2005 Nov; 4(11):705–711.

Being physically active in midlife could decrease a person's risk of dementia and Alzheimer's disease (AD) later in life. Individuals participating in leisure-time physical activity at least twice a week had a 60 percent lower odds of developing Alzheimer's disease compared to sedentary people (individuals participating in physical activity less than twice a week). The active group had 50 percent lower odds of developing dementia compared to the sedentary group.

Chen, H., Zhang, S.M., Schwarzschild, M.A., Hernán, M.A., Ascherio, A. Physical activity and the risk of Parkinson's disease. *Neurology* 2005 Feb 22; 64:664–669.

The Parkinson's study found that men who exercised regularly and vigorously early in their adult life lowered risk for Parkinson's by as much as 60 percent.

Christensen, H., Mackinnon, A. The association between mental, social and physical activity and cognitive performance in young and old subjects. *Age and Ageing* 1993; 22:175–182.

DiLorenzo, T.M., Bargman, E.P., Stucky-Ropp, R. et al. Long-term effects of aerobic exercise on psychological outcomes. *Preventative Medicine* 1999; 28:75–85.

Emery, C.F., Huppert, F.A., Schein, R.L. Relationships among age, exercise, health, and cognitive function in a British sample. *Gerontologist* 1995; 35:378–385.

Ferrucci, L., Izmirlian, G., Leveille, S. et al. Smoking, physical activity, and active life expectancy. *American Journal of Epidemiology* 1999: 149(7): 645–653.

Gomez-Pinilla, F., So, V., Kesslak, J.P. Spatial learning and physical activity contribute to the induction of fibroblast growth factor: neural substrates for increased cognition associated with exercise. *Neuroscience* 1998; 85:53–61.

Hakim, A.A., Petrovitch, H., Burchfiel, C.M. et al. Effects of walking on mortality among nonsmoking retired men. *New England Journal of Medicine* 1998; 338:94–99.

Hill, R.D., Storandt, M., Malley, M. The impact of long-term exercise training on psychological function in older adults. *Journal of Gerontology* 1993; 48:P12–17.

Kramer, A.F., Hahn, S., Cohen, N.J. et al. Ageing, fitness and neurocognitive function. *Nature* 1999; 400:418–419.

Laurin, D., Verreault, R., Lindsay, J., MacPherson, K., Rockwood, K. Physical activity and risk of cognitive impairment and dementia in elderly persons. *Archives of Neurology* 2001; 58:498–504.

Lee, I., Hsieh, C., Paffenbarger, R.S., Jr. Exercise intensity and longevity in men: the Harvard Alumni Health Study. *Journal of the American Medical Association* 1995; 273:1179–1184.

Mattson, M.P. Neuroprotective signaling and the aging brain: take away my food and let me run. *Brain Research* 2000; 886:47–53.

Neeper, S.A., Gomez-Pinilla, F., Choi, J., Cotman, C. Exercise and brain neurotrophins. *Nature* 1995; 373:109.

Okumiya, K., Matsubayashi, K., Wada, T. et al. Effects of exercise on neurobehavioral function in community-dwelling older people more than 75 years of age. *Journal of the American Geriatric Society* 1996; 44:569–572.

Pate, R.R., Pratt, M., Blair, S.H. et al. Physical activity and public health: a recommendation from the Centers for Disease Control and Prevention and the American College of Sports Medicine. *Journal of the American Medical Association* 1995; 273: 402–407.

Rogers, R.L., Meyer, J.S., Mortel, K.F. After reaching retirement age physical activity sustains cerebral perfusion and cognition. *Journal of the American Geriatric Society* 1990; 38:123–128.

Russo-Neustadt, A., Beard, R.C., Cotman, C.W. Exercise, antidepressant medications, and enhanced brain derived neurotrophic factor expression. *Neuropsychopharmacology* 1999; 21:679–682.

Salmon, P. Effects of physical exercise on anxiety, depression, and sensitivity to stress: a unifying theory. *Clinical Psychology* Review 2001; 21:33–61.

Scully, D., Kremer, J., Meade, M.M., Graham, R., Dudgeon, K. Physical exercise and psychological well being: a critical review. *British Journal of Sports Medicine* 1998; 32:111–120.

Shephard, R.J. What is the optimal type of physical activity to enhance health? *British Journal of Sports Medicine* 1997; 31:277–284.

Slaven, L., Lee, C. Mood and symptom reporting among middle-aged women: the relationship between menopausal status, hormone replacement therapy, and exercise participation. *Health Psychology: Official Journal of the Division of Health Psychology, American Psychological Association* 1997; 16:203–208.

Steinberg, H., Sykes, E.A., Moss, T. et al. Exercise enhances creativity independently of mood. *British Journal of Sports Medicine* 1997: 31:240–245.

U.S. Department of Health and Human Services. *Physical Activity and Health: A Report of the Surgeon General.* Atlanta, GA: U.S. Deparment of Health and Human Services, Centers for Disease Control and Prevention, National Center for Chronic Disease Prevention and Health Promotion 1996; 1–8, 85–172, 175–207.

Van Praag, H., Kempermann, G., Gage, F.H. Running increases cell proliferation and neurogenesis in the adult mouse dentate gyrus. *Nature Neuroscience* 1999; 2:266–270.

Exercise and Skin

Suominen, H., Heikkinen, E., Moisio, H., Viljamaa, K. Physical and chemical properties of skin in habitually trained and sedentary men. *British Journal of Dermatology* 1978 Aug; 99(2):147.

A number of physical and chemical properties of skin were examined in a study of twenty-nine habitually trained and twenty-nine sedentary men. Compared to the control group, the trained subjects had significantly higher values in the weights of skin samples of equal surface areas as well as the contents of hydroxyproline and nitrogen per skin surface area. When measured by a diaphragm method *in vivo*, the "elastic stiffness" (uncorrected for thickness) and "elastic efficiency" (the recovery of the deformation energy) of skin were significantly higher in the trained men compared to those in the untrained men. The results suggest that skin reflects the adaptation to habitual endurance training by increasing its mass and strengthening its structure. The study did not, however, reveal any differences between physically active and sedentary men in changes due to biological aging.

Diet and Mortality

Kant, A.K., Graubard, B.I., Schatzkin, A. Dietary patterns predict mortality in a national cohort: The national health interview surveys, 1987 and 1992. *Journal of Nutrition* 2004; 134:1793–1799.

There is a growing body of evidence that demonstrates that following a diet that complies with the Dietary Guidelines may reduce the risk of chronic disease. Recently, it was reported that dietary patterns consistent with recommended dietary guidance were associated with a lower risk of mortality among individuals age forty-five years and older in the United States. The authors of the study estimated that about 16 percent and 9 percent of mortality from any cause in men and women, respectively, could be eliminated by the adoption of desirable dietary behaviors.

Exercise and Dental Health

Al-Zahrani, M.S., Borawski, E.A., Bissada, N.F. Periodontitis and three health-enhancing behaviors: maintaining normal weight, engaging in recommended level of exercise and consuming a high-quality diet. *Journal of Periodontology* 2005 Aug; 76(8):1362–1366.

Individuals who exercised and had healthy eating habits and maintained a normal weight were 40 percent less likely to develop periodontitis, a gum infection that can result in loss of teeth.

Exercise and Hearing

Hutchinson, K., Alessio, H., Dichiara, J., Crain, T. Study finds higher cardiovascular fitness associated with greater hearing acuity. *The Hearing Journal* 2002; 55(8):32.

Hearing is regulated by one's health, which is largely within our control. Among other aspects of health, maintaining a healthy cardiovascular system through regular exercise can lessen the effects of aging on the hearing processes, thus preventing decreases in hearing ability and maintaining hearing levels over time ... cardiovascular fitness contributes to better neural integrity in the cochlea, specifically the outer hair cells, by ensuring ample supplies of oxygen-rich blood to surrounding organs. Another possible explanation is that people who are heart healthy maintain overall health better, thus limiting damage to hearing due to noise exposure, medications, and disease.

index